A Clinician's Guide to
Non-Pharmacological
Dementia Therapies

of related interest

Sensory Modulation in Dementia Care
Assessment and Activities for Sensory-Enriched Care
Tina Champagne
ISBN 978 1 78592 733 1
eISBN 978 1 78450 427 4

Essentials of Dementia
Everything You Really Need to Know for Working in Dementia Care
Dr Shibley Rahman and Professor Rob Howard
ISBN 978 1 78592 397 5
eISBN 978 1 78450 754 1

Understanding Behaviour in Dementia
that Challenges, Second Edition
A Guide to Assessment and Treatment
Ian Andrew James and Louisa Jackman
ISBN 978 1 78592 264 0
eISBN 978 1 78450 551 6

Enhancing Health and Wellbeing in Dementia
A Person-Centred Integrated Care Approach
Dr Shibley Rahman
Forewords by Professor Sube Banerjee and Lisa Rodrigues
ISBN 978 1 78592 037 0
eISBN 978 1 78450 291 1

Cognitive Behavioural Therapy With Older People
Interventions for Those With and Without Dementia
Ian Andrew James
ISBN 978 1 84905 100 2
eISBN 978 0 85700 283 9

A Clinician's Guide to Non-Pharmacological Dementia Therapies

Dr Daniel J. Nightingale

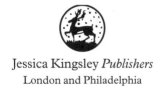

Jessica Kingsley *Publishers*
London and Philadelphia

First published in 2019
by Jessica Kingsley Publishers
73 Collier Street
London N1 9BE, UK
and
400 Market Street, Suite 400
Philadelphia, PA 19106, USA

www.jkp.com

Library of Congress Cataloging in Publication Data
A CIP catalog record for this book is available from the Library of Congress

British Library Cataloguing in Publication Data
A CIP catalogue record for this book is available from the British Library

ISBN 978 1 78592 595 5
eISBN 978 1 78592 602 0

Printed and bound in Great Britain

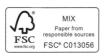

Contents

Acknowledgments

I have often been encouraged to write a book on this topic, and much encouragement has come from one of my closest friends and colleagues Dr Simon Duff. Therefore, thank you for your friendship, brotherhood, encouragement, support and, of course, kebabs!

Sue Ashcroft, you are the reason I became a dementia specialist in the first place. I'm sure you recall how all that unfolded back at Knowsley Manor in Liverpool! Joan Clarke (my adopted mother), you are the reason for me getting to where I've got – wherever that is. Your tireless efforts to promote me, and more importantly, my work, will never be forgotten. Ellen Poynton has been a part of my life for many years, as has Gary Fitzgerald. You have both been brilliant, and without you so many opportunities and doors would never have been opened in the first place. Drs David and Karen Daugherty, your love and friendship mean more than I can ever express, as does that of Patrick and Sylvia Baize and the Chino Valley Mennonite community.

Then there is Dr Umesh Tiwari, my twin brother from another mother from California (not sure how that works, but it just does!). Not only are you an amazing physician and clinical hypnotherapist, you are also a true role model of professionalism. Just as an aside, I think you are also a great dad to your son and amazing husband to your beautiful wife.

I have been inspired by all of you – and many more clinicians and friends – to write such things as *My Dreams of Being* and *My Dreams of Being: Inclusion of Reality*, which is being used around the world to improve the quality of life of people living through the challenges of neurocognitive disorders.

I also owe great thanks to Sarah Murdoch, editor-in-chief at *Expert Care Manager Journal*, who has believed in me and my writing for a few years. At the time of writing this book, Sarah has published my work in 17 copies of the journal, with more to come. Thank you for helping me to educate your readers.

Also, my son Kieran is forever saying how proud he is of me, so this is dedicated to you and my daughter Sladjana.

Back in February 2018, I spent about 5 weeks with the best nephew anyone could ever wish for. He and his wife Sarah played a huge part in my decision to write this book, so it is also for you.

It would be remiss of me not to thank my commissioning editor Andrew James, whose patience and tolerance knows no bounds! Finally, thank you to everyone I have known, and met, throughout the world – as a colleague, patient or client – during my years as a clinical dementia specialist, dementia consultant, general psychotherapist, stand-up comedian and actor. You have all played a part and my gratitude is extended to each and every one of you.

Dr Daniel J. Nightingale

Introduction

I have been in the care profession since the age of 14 when I became a volunteer at my local charity for children and adults with learning disabilities. It was called the Peter Pan Club. However, prior to that, I remember being in hospital at around the age of 6 or 7, so it was in the early 1970s. I don't recall the reason for my hospitalization and my folks are no longer around to ask. However, there was a boy of a similar age in the next bed to me. He had no arms, was unable to speak and looked very scared. He got no visitors, so I assumed he had no parents, or no parents who cared. The nurses and doctors were silent around his bed, and yet when they were with me they talked and smiled. My parents visited regularly. I would sneak out of my bed and take some toys for him to play with. One day he was taken away and I never saw him again. As I reflect, this was my first lesson in how *not* to care.

At the age of 53 – where on earth have those years gone? – I remain in the care profession, and each day I continue to learn *how* to care. By this I mean truly engaging with my patients and empathizing with them on many levels, accepting their individuality and personality constructs. As a student I learned about everything from disease to hygiene; my world consisted of clinical books, research books, lectures and classes. However, it wasn't until I was interacting with people that I learned how different people were. They didn't fit into a "category" and they couldn't be explained by a "syndrome." This is because people are as individual as a fingerprint and must be treated as such. I believe people like Patch Adams, Abraham Maslow and Tom Kitwood understood this, hence the positive impact they have had in medicine and psychology.

Throughout the years I have had the opportunity to develop models, approaches and interventions that have had, and continue to have, a positive impact on the people I serve.

This book is a combination of all the skills, knowledge and tools I have developed as a clinician, researcher, educator, journal writer, author, stand-up comedian and actor. Wherever possible I use the diagnostic term of "neurocognitive disorder" as defined in the Diagnostic and Statistical Manual of Mental Disorders, fifth edition (DSM-5; APA 2013). However, for ease of reading I also refer to cognitive change and dementia.

Here is a quotation from Dr Patch Adams, by whom I am fortunate enough to have been taught: "The purpose of any doctor or any human in general should not be to simply delay the death of the patient, but to increase the person's quality of life." He also said that "The most radical act anyone can commit is to be happy."

It is this inspiration that motivates me to do what I do. For this I will be eternally grateful because each time I turn a frown into a smile I have accomplished my goal, and this is what the book is about.

Currently, there is no cure for any of the primary dementias. Researchers from different fields and disciplines around the world are working frantically to change that. As they do so, it is our job to offer therapies that serve to improve quality of life to such an extent that people with a diagnosis of Alzheimer's disease or other neurocognitive disorder may live as well as possible through their unique journeys.

Through the use of case studies I have described and discussed how various therapies such as cognitive behavior therapy, neuro linguistic programming and hypno-psychotherapy can help achieve an improved quality of life for the people we support. Also described are the models within which we can use these therapies, and a strategy for reducing the negative effects of transitional shock that may present before, during or after a major change to an individual's life.

Chapter 2 describes an intervention called DTS-VADRA2016. The focus of this intervention is on a strategy aimed at identifying an individual's risk of developing vascular dementia and Alzheimer's disease in order that a program can be developed and implemented to reduce those risks. Appendix 2 in Chapter 10 can be downloaded from www.jkp.com/catalogue/book/9781785925955.

There are a number of rare forms of neurocognitive disorders that affect both adults and children. In Chapter 12 I discuss some therapies and interventions that can be used with this client group.

If you are a clinician I believe you will find the book of great value in your practice. For everyone else, I am sure you will also find value in part, or even the whole of the book, and that it will serve its purpose well.

Chapter 1

The Nightingale Model of Psycho-Social Support

According to Alzheimer's Disease International, someone in the world develops dementia every 3 seconds. Each and every one of those people is individual in their character, personality and psychological construct. By many this is seen as a problem, but to a clinician problems should only ever be seen as solutions in disguise. Therefore, to uncover those solutions, it is necessary to have a model that is useful to both clinician and the person living with a diagnosis(es) of dementia.

The Nightingale Model of Psycho-Social Support is currently being used in a number of practices by a wide range of clinicians associated with Dementia Therapy Specialists throughout the UK and US (Figure 1.1). This is a true person centered approach developed over my many years of clinical practice. Though there are many models available in the world of psychiatry, psychology and psychotherapy, this model is much easier to apply and more comprehensible to someone experiencing cognitive change. It is a structured process that can be used by any professional, in any setting, who is supporting an individual and, where appropriate, his or her family through their unique journey of dementia. The value to using this model is that it has been developed to be fully inclusive of everyone involved in that journey. We must always place the individual at the center of any support we provide, and this model achieves that goal.

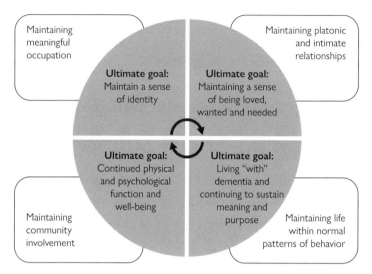

Figure 1.1 The Nightingale Model of Psycho-Social support

Increased value is added to this model as it was developed following consultation with 20 people living with dementia and their immediate caregivers or family members. The four outer areas were considered by them to be important in order to be empowered enough that their journey was as positive and meaningful as possible. The four inner quadrants are their ultimate goals that avoid malignant social psychology.

Using a case study, I will explain how this model works and the positive impact it has had on one gentleman, his wife and their quality of life.

CASE STUDY

Martin was 74 years old when he was diagnosed with a mixed neurocognitive disorder (NCD) of both frontotemporal and vascular dementia. At the time of diagnosis in the summer of 2016 Martin lived at home with his wife Janet, who was 68. However, when Martin was referred to me he was living in a care home due to behavioral and psychological changes that had brought many challenges, including social withdrawal, and verbal and physical aggression toward a number of professionals and family members, including Janet. The care home is specifically set up to support people like Martin and it was they who referred him to me. The move was intended to be temporary in the hope that Martin's behavioral and psychological symptoms could be managed sufficiently for him to return home.

On meeting Martin I was struck by how intelligent he was and how active he likes to be. However, it also struck me that his current environment was contributing to his ever-increasing agitation and frustration. Through discussion with Martin and Janet I was able to build a solid profile about their likes and dislikes, about their relationship and about their expectations moving forward. Initially, after moving in to the care home, Martin would go home at the weekends and spend time with Janet. A dedicated member of the care home team was always available to go out and provide any support necessary if he became aggressive in any way. For the first few months this worked perfectly. Then it began to change and Janet was no longer able to live with his lability of mood. There was resistance from the family to using any kind of medication, thus I turned to the model of psycho-social support. Through the approach of Shared Action Planning, which put both Martin and Janet at the center of this model, the following plan was created.

The starting point is always one of prioritizing the challenges. After discussing the four outer and inner quadrant areas, *maintaining meaningful occupation with the ultimate goal of being able to maintain a sense of identity* was established by both Martin and Janet as the number one priority. This was selected as, prior to retirement at the age of 65, Martin had been the headmaster of a very large private school, holding huge responsibility including budgetary management and a leadership role. In addition, he was a professor of history. There was a feeling that this identity was now slipping away and that his personhood and sense of well-being were now undermined. In effect, he was experiencing malignant social psychology, and this was impacting negatively on every aspect of his life and relationships. Martin was challenged more by changes to his personality and character than he was by cognitive change. Socially inappropriate behavior, a lack of inhibition and frequent mood changes were the areas that caused the most difficulties by affecting Martin's quality of life. Ultimately, these challenges impacted negatively on both Martin and Janet's leisure and social interactions and their relationship with each other. Negative thoughts and actions became the norm as Martin continued to succumb to his journey.

Agreed Action

Martin had a very good friend who was also a professor of history. He was much younger and not yet retired. This friend, Professor Matthews, agreed to be part of Martin and Janet's plan and agreed to support him, once a week, in running a history class at the care home. This would become part of the daily social activity program for residents and it was billed as Professor Martin Anton's Modern History Lectures. Each week, a different topic would be chosen by Martin, with the lectures delivered every Wednesday afternoon at 2pm.

Outcome

This action achieved many things for Martin, who requested to be referred to as Professor Anton. This gave back his identity. Not only did it help him regain, and maintain, a sense of identity and self-worth, but it increased his self-esteem and confidence too. The necessity for him to plan each lecture led to his mind and thoughts being focused on the positive behavior of lesson planning and lecture presentation notes. There was a spring in his step again. His friend and former colleague Professor Matthews would call in two nights a week to offer his valuable input as his collaborator, and Janet would also give a supporting hand during her daily visits. Within a few days we began to see a change in the professor's behavior. His body language was also notably changing to one of positivity. He was smiling more, engaging with people through conversation and he insisted on wearing a suit once more. There was no time to focus on his challenges, though he did become irritable on occasion. However, those occasional irritable outbursts were easily managed by engaging with him about modern history and watching a short video about his chosen Wednesday topic. From that moment on, Professor Martin Anton was addressed as such by the care home staff and visiting professionals, unless he asked them to address him as Martin.

As the change in the professor's behavior became more apparent, 2 weeks later we addressed the second priority that was identified by the couple. This was *maintaining platonic and intimate relationships with the ultimate goal of maintaining a sense of feeling loved, wanted and needed*. Very often with frontotemporal dementia we see the person lose their ability to display empathy, but this was not the case with him. Somehow, this remained intact, which meant that I was able to have an open, honest and frank conversation about this part of the model and how it would help with this particular challenge.

Since the first priority was addressed and implemented, Professor Anton had started to spend more time engaging with the people in his immediate environment; he even began a friendship with Alvin, a fellow resident who had a huge interest in history and who had attended both lectures to date. That relationship was evolving and he was once again growing closer to Professor Matthews. These relationships were to be nurtured and encouraged in order for them to develop as much as possible. We were now able to turn our attention to the couple's intimate relationship.

Up until Professor Anton was diagnosed with dementia, he and Janet had enjoyed a healthy, fulfilling intimate relationship, would always hold hands and snuggle together both on the sofa and in bed. The day the diagnosis was delivered, he became cold toward his wife, withdrew from any intimacy with her and refused to discuss it. He even moved himself into one of the guest bedrooms. There is a great deal of stigma around sexual fulfillment, sexual behavior and intimate relationships for people who are living with dementia and this can lead to a further reduction in quality of life. Neither one of them had raised this issue in the past but Janet felt confident enough in our relationship that she could now broach the subject. She was still in love with her husband and she continued to love him every waking moment of her life. Not to have him touch or hold her was devastating and caused her a great deal of emotional anguish and pain. Once Janet began to open up about her feelings, a tear was observed falling down Professor Anton's cheek. This was validation that he continued to empathize with his wife through emotional empathy, sometimes referred to as affective or primitive empathy. This is a subjective state that results from emotional contagion and happens automatically, usually at an unconscious level.

Through exploration, using person centered counseling, it became apparent that Professor Anton had spent a great deal of time over the last 12 months feeling unwanted and unneeded by his wife, and when the decision was made for him to move into a care home he felt completely and totally unloved and rejected. When he was told that he had dementia his self-confidence, self-esteem and self-worth received a massive hit and, for that reason, his usual extrovert character adopted the opposite persona of introvert, leading him to reject everyone, including Janet. So, at this point they both agreed that they wanted to reinstate their intimate relationship and that they would make an attempt at a weekend visit to their home. Before Janet left him that day, they hugged each other. It had been their first real closeness in quite some time.

Agreed Action

A weekend visit was arranged where Professor Anton and Janet would spend time together, with a dedicated member of the care home team accessible to visit if necessary. This gave both Professor Anton and his wife something additional to look forward too, and they both stated they were excited about their "date."

Outcome

The following Monday I visited the couple at the care home to discuss how things went. There had been no need for any form of crisis intervention from the support team and they had enjoyed their weekend. They had been intimate in the way they had in the past and Professor Anton's behavior was now more socially acceptable and he was much less aggressive with those around him. I felt it important to have regular 1:1 consults with him and to address any concerns he had as they emerged. A new care plan was developed for further weekend home visits. At Professor Anton's request, these home visits were agreed as every 2 weeks.

Through the use of this model we are seeing a positive impact in the quality of life of Professor and Mrs Anton. No longer is the dementia the main focus. We have been able to shift that focus back to the positive, meaningful and engaging activities that have defined his personality and character for many years. There has been no need for antipsychotic medicines and he has not been taking acetylcholinesterase inhibitors. His cognition appears to be stable at this point and, though he sometimes struggles to find the right words or phrases, his speech and language remain unaffected by dysphasia. So far, we have supported Professor Anton to re-establish his identity as a professor, friend, husband and lover. Once again he is beginning to feel loved, wanted and needed, and we are able to demonstrate that the behavioral and psychological symptoms of dementia cannot always be attributed to the change in brain pathology of someone with an NCD. Instead, we begin to see that it is our attitudes, approaches and belief systems that do this and that they need to be challenged and changed. As I continue to support Professor Anton and Janet through this model, we turn our attention to their third priority of *maintaining community involvement with the ultimate aim of continued physical and psychological well-being*. They both agreed that we could continue to build on Professor Anton's newfound belief that he still has something of value to contribute not only to his local community, but to society as a whole.

Now we start looking at Professor Anton's existing skills, abilities, competencies and interests in his local community (i.e. the care home) and the society as a whole (i.e. his external environment). We know about his obvious interest in history, but what is there outside of that? He has now grown in confidence and his self-esteem continues to increase. He is physically fit and active and was once a member of the local badminton club. We discussed the possibility of him going to visit the club to catch up with friends and fellow badminton players. Reluctant at first, he spent time with his wife looking at some photographs of that aspect of his life. This appeared to reignite his interest to a degree that he decided it might be a good idea to go and visit the club. He was empowered to make this informed choice while being enabled and supported by his allocated key worker at the care home to make the necessary arrangements.

The aim of this model is to avoid any type of malignant social psychology. In order to achieve this, individuals require continued support, consistency in approach and the development of valued, trusted relationships with those supporting them along their unique journey. I am a part of the journey of all the people I support, as are many other professionals and informal caregivers. We all have a role to play in avoiding the onset of any kind of malignancy, which is why this model must be incorporated as part of an overall care plan. Therefore, *maintaining community involvement* is crucial to an individual's sense of self. By nature we are social animals – very few of us choose to isolate ourselves from our fellow man, but it is a common behavior adopted by many people once they move into a care home. There are two reasons for this. First, in some care homes tasks become far more important than human interaction, which then leads to residents becoming "invisible" to those around them. Second, there is an attitude of self-preservation that is adopted by many people who move in to a care home – through choice they become withdrawn and isolate themselves. Maintaining community involvement should always be part of the individual's overall care and, for Professor Anton, there were many benefits.

Agreed Action

Professor Anton agreed to call Kelly, the secretary of the badminton club. They have known each other for many years but it had been almost 2 years since they last spoke. He was to be supported by his key worker in doing this. A date was to be arranged for him to go and meet with Kelly, have spot of lunch and talk about reinstating his membership. The aim here is to ensure continued physical and psychological function and well-being, with an underlying goal of ensuring he has positive activities to consider and relationships to form. If people living with dementia have a purpose to getting up in the morning then their motivation improves greatly. Just like everyone else, they continue to feel valued and this model takes that fact into consideration.

Outcome

The agreed action was carried through and Professor Anton went to meet Kelly with his wife Janet. It transpired that before he began to develop the symptoms of dementia he was going to join the committee. One of the things he had spoken to me about during our 1:1 consults was how much he missed "life." Once he moved into the care home he felt his "life" was over.

These negative thoughts had fueled his feelings of worthlessness and led him down the road of depression. Until we started to work together and before the introduction of this psycho-social model, Professor Anton had, to all intents and purposes, given up. As the model is being implemented exactly how it should be, to meet the unique and individual needs of this particular person, his own mindset had shifted. He began to realize that he was living a life that dementia wanted him to lead. His own knowledge and beliefs around this disease were now being challenged and he was beginning to take control of "it" as opposed to "it" taking control of him. During his visit they discussed ways in which he could have input as a committee member and it was agreed that, with some support from other committee members, this could be facilitated.

During my next visit to see Professor Anton it was clear that he continued to grow and develop as a human being. His particular dementia was no longer defining who he was to become. Instead, he was making those decisions. I often quote Carl Jung, who once said that an individual is a "unique, dynamic, ever changing self." This is relevant to each and every one of us.

We can see that this model is having a very positive impact on improving quality of life. Professor Anton's relationship with his wife is now in a good place and there are many smiles where there were once only frowns. My therapeutic relationship with the couple was based on honesty, openness and genuineness. As such, we were now able to proceed to the final quadrant in the model: *maintaining life within normal patterns of behavior with the ultimate goal of living "with" dementia and continuing to sustain meaning and purpose.* As we have seen, Professor Anton is now spending weekends back home, he is delivering weekly lectures with support and has become a member of the badminton club's committee. The next stage is maintaining this for as long as possible within the parameters of his type of dementia.

Agreed Action

For Professor Anton and Janet, "normal patterns of behavior" referred to a life that was as peaceful and constant as possible for as long as they are on their journey through dementia. They agreed that the time had come for him to return home once again, where I would visit weekly and the crisis intervention team, attached to the care home, would remain accessible should they be needed. Neither of them wanted to consider having to use any medicines, such as risperidone, aimed at managing behavioral challenges. However, both agreed and understood that at some point along the journey, this might have to be reviewed. For now, this model was proving fruitful.

Outcome

Four weeks after Professor Anton returned home, we pulled all elements of this model together and reviewed the overall outcome and impact that was leading to a current *maintenance of a life within normal patterns of behavior* for both him and his wife.

He continues to deliver his Wednesday afternoon History lectures at the care home and his work on the committee at the badminton club. Both platonic friendships and his intimate relationship with Janet continue to be held together, and once a week I make my clinical visits to evaluate all aspects of his care and support.

At the time of writing, he remains free of medicine and has developed various other tools to help manage any behavioral challenges that emerge day to day. As you read further into this book you will learn about some of those tools.

In summary, this model has had a very positive impact in this case, as it has done in many other clinical cases. A change of mindset by professionals and people living with dementia is an essential element if we are to get the best out of this model. Although clinically, we see all NCDs as neurodegenerative in nature, a true person centered approach will always lead to an increased quality of life, thus resulting in a more positive clinical outcome.

Chapter 2

The DTS-VADRA2016

Before discussing the DTS-VADRA2016 tool, and demonstrating its use through a clinical case study, I would like to briefly discuss vascular neurocognitive disorder (vascular NCD), which is regarded as the second most common type of dementia after Alzheimer's disease. However, mixed NCDs of both the Alzheimer and vascular type are common. Exact prevalence rates are not known but we believe them to be more common than was previously thought. This has been demonstrated through autopsies.

The word dementia (a negative term that, as a diagnosis, is now replaced by the term neurocognitive disorder) has its grounding in Latin and means madness. It describes a set of symptoms that can include memory loss and difficulties with thinking, problem solving or language. In vascular NCD, these symptoms occur when the brain is damaged because of problems with the supply of blood to the brain.

A Reminder of Causes

Vascular NCD is caused by reduced blood supply to the brain due to diseased blood vessels.

To be healthy and function properly, brain cells need a constant supply of blood to bring oxygen and nutrients. Blood is delivered to the brain through a network of vessels called the vascular system. If the vascular system within the brain becomes damaged – so that the blood vessels leak or become blocked – then blood cannot reach the brain cells and they will eventually die.

This death of brain cells can cause problems with memory, thinking or reasoning. Together these three elements are known as cognition. When these cognitive problems are bad enough to have a significant impact on daily life, this is known as vascular NCD.

This type of NCD is a lifestyle disease and therefore something we can reduce the risk of developing. *That's the good news!* Now for the *really good news*: there is now evidence that suggests the neuritic plaques and tangles symptomatic of Alzheimer's disease can lay dormant in the brain and only manifest when the brain is damaged through tiny little strokes referred to as transient ischemic attacks (TIAs). It is these TIAs that lead to vascular NCD. This could explain why mixed dementia, living with both vascular NCD and NCD due to Alzheimer's disease, is very common. This evidence came to light during the Nun Study of Aging and Alzheimer's disease, whose founding investigator was David Snowdon (2001). This research originated at the University of Minnesota, but later moved to the University of Kentucky. Following the retirement of David Snowdon, the study returned to Minnesota and remains ongoing as a longitudinal study.

This means, if we do all we can to adopt a healthy lifestyle, we are making every effort to reduce our risk of developing not just vascular NCD, but also NCD due to Alzheimer's disease.

What is the DTS-VADRA2016?

Currently, and for the foreseeable future, there is no cure for any of the primary NCDs such as NCD due to Alzheimer's disease, vascular NCD and NCD with Lewy bodies, and there lies our challenge as clinicians practicing in this very complex field.

For this reason, our current focus must be on reducing the risk of developing it through prevention wherever possible. There is a common misconception that dementia only affects seniors, but in today's modern world we know this to be untrue. For example, 1 in 150,000 children are born with a form of dementia called Niemen–Pick type C. In the UK, there are approximately 43,000 people with young onset dementia and in the US this figure stands at approximately 200,000. Niemann–Pick UK (NPUK) estimate a prevalence of 1 in 120,000, with some recent evidence suggesting this may be an underestimate.

Many of those diagnosed with young onset dementia are aged between 40 and 50, therefore a number of them are working age with young families to support, mortgages and rents to pay and other responsibilities typical of that age group.

With regard to vascular NCD, this is a lifestyle disease, and by adopting a healthy lifestyle we can reduce our risk of developing it. If the evidence gleamed from the Nun Study is correct, we can therefore reduce our risk of triggering the symptoms of Alzheimer's disease too.

The message we must get across to society is that it is imperative for people to take responsibility for their own good health and well-being, both physical and psychological.

With this in mind I have developed the Dementia Therapy Specialists Vascular Dementia Risk Assessment 2016 (DTS-VADRA2016), which is useful in three key areas:

1. It identifies an individual's risk of developing vascular NCD (low, medium, high).

The benefits of identifying an individual's risk of developing vascular NCD include the following:

- It provides an awareness of where those risks come from. For example, are they due to lifestyle, underlying pathology of existing disease or heredity factors? Gathering those data is the starting point to making this model effective.

- It offers the option of being proactive in taking steps to completely remove those risks or maintain them at the lowest level possible.

- It empowers the individual to take full responsibility for their physical and psychological health and well-being ahead of any need for reactive medical or psychological intervention.

2. A Shared Action Plan (SAP) is developed that is aimed at greatly reducing those risks and promoting physical and psychological well-being.

There are many benefits to a SAP, which include:

- Enabling the individual to be at the center of the plan, to be the key driver and operator with responsibility and accountability for it.

- A structured support system from the clinician that serves to encourage, motivate and enable the individual to achieve the set goals.

- The plan can involve family members, friends and fellow professionals selected by that person.

- The individual has a copy of the SAP and can take it whenever they visit a professional. At the end of the visit, that professional can write in it so that everyone remains informed.

3. Supporting an individual who has the earliest stages of vascular NCD in reducing rapid deterioration and further cognitive dysfunction.

If our client presents with early onset dementia, we have an excellent opportunity to use this model to have a direct impact on slowing down its progress. The benefits here include:

- Positive symptomatic management through non-pharmacological strategies.

- An opportunity to support the individual to change their mindset from negative to positive if required.

- An opportunity to educate the client and encourage them to take control of their cognitive change (it may be that the model of psycho-social support we covered in Chapter 1 will also be used at this stage).

The DTS-VADRA2016

Each question relates to lifestyle. The score is (1) no/low risk; (2) medium risk; or (3) high risk.

Final outcomes will be calculated as no/low risk, medium risk or high risk of developing vascular NCD by adding up the numbers in each column. The column with the greatest number equates to level of risk.

On conclusion, the appropriate advice and guidance will be given with a SAP and a treatment/therapy plan if indicated.

The DTS-VADRA2016 that follows will be completed and plans formulated by taking the data from a case study of an existing client. The client, whom I will call Mr Adams, was referred to me by his GP after he diagnosed him with type 2 diabetes (previously known as non-insulin dependent diabetes mellitus, or NIDDM). He was 59 years of age, married with two sons aged 23 and 25, and was employed at the local crematorium where he had worked for over 30 years. Mr Adams had a wide circle of friends and, as such, a very active social life. He planned to retire in

9 months' time when he reached his 60th birthday and travel through Europe, the US and Canada. His wife had retired from the police force when she was 55. Financially set, they were busy preparing to embark on their new adventure. The diagnosis had come as a shock to Mr Adams so he sought help and support to lessen its impact.

We discussed looking at the level of risk posed to him in relation to diabetic dementia. A number of studies have demonstrated that type 2 diabetes in midlife is associated with increased risk of developing both NCD due to Alzheimer's disease and vascular NCD. One piece of research is known as the Rotterdam Study, which was published in *Diabetalogia* back in 1999 (Ott et al. 1996). Their outcomes demonstrated that the presence of diabetes almost doubled the risk of NCDs, and those being treated with insulin (which, at this point, Mr Adams was not) were at an even greater risk. It is relevant to point out that type 2 diabetes often develops into type 1, which was previously known as insulin dependent diabetes, or IDD.

In relation to this case, we agreed on two key objectives. These were:

1. To consider current lifestyle and identify necessary changes that would prevent Mr Adams' type 2 diabetes from developing into type 1.

2. Develop a strategy that would ensure his blood glucose levels were kept within normal parameters.

You will see Mr Adams' completed DTS-VADRA2016 in Table 2.1; the advice offered in Box 2.1; the Pre Shared Action Plan Inter-related Cycle of Priorities in Figure 2.1; the SAP in Box 2.2; and the Current Inter-related Cycle of Priorities in Figure 2.2.

Table 2.1 Completed DTS-VADRA2016

Name: Mr Trevor Adams

DOB: 12/31/1959

Address: 14 Trees Lane, Treetown, Tree TR1 TRE

Telephone and Email: 00700700700 TA.AD133@treetown.com

Date of Assessment: 3/27/2018

Name of Assessor: Dr D.J. Nightingale

Name and Contact Details of Primary Physician/GP: Dr Greentree, Greentree Practice, Greentree Avenue, Greentree TR2 TRE. Tel: 42325232

Question	Answer	No to low	Medium	High
Male/female?	M	1		
Age?	59.3	1		
Occupation?	Crematorium operator	1		
Family history?	No history of dementia	1		
Hypertension? 126/86 at time of consult today	Yes, but only slightly. No medication (Rx) but weight loss advice given by GP		2	
History of heart disease?	Mother died as a result of a ruptured aortic aneurism			3
Married?	Yes	1		
Current diagnosis(es)?	Elevated blood pressure, type 2 Diabetes, obesity			3
Current medical treatment?	No medication Rx as yet. Weekly monitoring and observation at diabetes clinic	1		

cont.

Question	Answer	No to low	Medium	High
Smoker? How many a day?	Yes – a 20-pack a day			3
Units of alcohol intake each week?	42 units – he drinks, on average, 2 pints of lager each night. The recommended amount is 14 units per week			3
How do you manage your stress?	Emotionally eat, smoke, watch TV			3
Level of education?	High school with no further formal education			3
Any deficits in attention and executive function?	None apparent at this time	1		
Any memory loss? If so, what type? Regularity? Frequency?	Though he reports working memory deficit, no evidence of this on the MMSE	1		
MMSE score?	30	1		
Blood pressure reading?	126/86		0 (already scored above)	
Current diet and weight?	High-carb, high-sugar diet Diagnosed as obese by GP at a weight of 250 lb and a height of 5 ft. 10 in. = BMI 35.9 He needs to lose 100 lb			3
Evidence of ear creases?	Yes			3

When last screened for diabetes?	1 week ago Diagnosed with type 2 diabetes			3 (though already scored, the necessity to be tested is scored)
Any anticholinergic drugs prescribed such as Benadryl, Tylenol, antidepressants? UTI medication? If so, what and why?	No	1		
Do you take a Vitamin D supplement? (4000 IU per day as a supplement)	No		2	
Do you regularly take heartburn meds? (e.g. Prilosec, Prevacid)	No	1		

MMSE, Mini-Mental State Examination; Rx, prescription UTI, urinary tract infection

Overall Risk, Advice, Wheel of Balance and SAP

The overall risk for this individual is 27 = High.

BOX 2.1 ADVICE OFFERED

With the aim of reducing the risk of Mr Adams developing an NCD, the following advice was presented to him:

- A need to lose 100 lb (45.36 kg).

- A need to review current diet.

- A need to stop smoking and drinking excess alcohol.

- A need for a minimum of 20 minutes of cardiovascular exercise three times a week.

- A need to address underlying emotional issues through appropriate therapy.

- A need to develop appropriate, healthy stress management strategies.

- Evaluate cognitive function monthly through Mini-Mental State Examination (MMSE) and Saint Louis University Mental Status (SLUMS) evaluations.

- A need to create a post-retirement vision board.

- A need to set goals as part of a SAP.

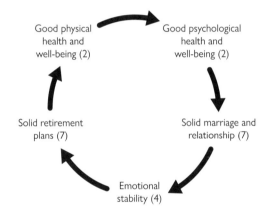

Figure 2.1 Pre Shared Action Plan Inter-related Cycle of Priorities

Mr Adams chose these five areas as his priorities in life and scored each of the above between 0 and 10, with 0 being the worst place he could be and 10 the healthiest. As you can see, he allocated a score of 2 to both his good physical and psychological health and well-being, a 4 for his emotional stability, and 7 for his marriage and relationship and retirement plans. This was useful in assisting with creating his SAP.

BOX 2.2 AGREED SHARED ACTION PLAN

Mr Adams was motivated to make the necessary changes for the following reasons:

1. To avoid developing an NCD.

2. To improve his overall health and well-being.

3. To enjoy a long, healthy retirement with his wife.

He involved his wife as part of his SAP and agreed to work with me in therapy. The following goals were set.

Short-term goals

- To develop a healthy eating program.

- To lose weight in a timely manner.

- To plan a post-retirement trip.

- To create a vision board.

- To enter therapy.

Long-term goals

- To stop smoking and drinking excessive amounts of alcohol.

- To maintain blood glucose levels within normal parameters of between 72 and 108 mg/dl.

- Resolve underlying emotional issues.

- Have no cognitive decline.

- Have a great retirement.

Plan

1. Mr Adams to change his nutritional intake to that of a Mediterranean diet – advice was given to him about what this constitutes. It is high in monounsaturated fat, which has been shown by countless studies to lower the risk

of heart disease, cognitive decline, Alzheimer's disease, cancer and depression. One such well-known Spanish study, whose principal investigators were R. Estruch and M.A. Martinez-Gonzalez, is the PREDIMED study (this stands for Prevencion con Dieta Mediterranea, or Prevention with Mediterranean Diet) (Estruch et al. 2013). For Mr Adams, this means an introduction of fruit and vegetables, grains and protein foods. Though wholewheat bread is part of the Mediterranean diet, Mr Adams was advised to drop bread from his diet, along with beer, soda and other high-sugar foods. The aim was to lose a minimum of 2 lb (0.9 kg) per week and a maximum of 4 lb (1.8 kg) per week. A photo of himself as a slimmer man will be posted onto his vision board.

2. Mr Adams will sit down with his wife and plan their future trip. Setting target dates will assist with his focus, and a picture of each place to be visited will be posted onto his vision board.

3. The final part of this SAP is for Mr Adams to enter therapy with the aim of resolving underlying emotional issues. The goals set in therapy are:

    i.   Uncover the emotional issues that, following spotlighting, appear to be at the unconscious level.

    ii. Develop a therapy plan to address the issues uncovered.

    iii. To help develop a smoking cessation program.

    iv. Mr Adams to learn how to use various psychological tools that will ensure he is equipped with coping skills and strategies to manage any future stresses.

Signed: _____

                                                   Clinician

Signed: _____

                                                     Client

Progress

At the time of writing, Mr Adams' journey continues in a positive way. We are 3 months in to his SAP and he has lost 32 lb (14.5 kg). This is just under a third of the set target suggested by his GP. He has taken up a daily walking routine and is going to attend yoga classes with his wife. Following one session of hypnotherapy Mr Adams quit smoking (hypnotherapy has a 79% success rate for smoking cessation).

At the end of a spotlighting session, the chosen therapy was an eclectic approach of hypnosis to uncover emotional issues and reinforce the absence of the need to smoke cigarettes; hypno-psychotherapy with the aim of helping Mr Adams to let go of any negative experiences; and cognitive behavior therapy with neuro linguistic programming to alter any negative thoughts and images so they become positive. After weekly sessions for the past 6 weeks, Mr Adams has made great strides and is now more in control of his life.

In later chapters in this book we will be looking at these therapies, and their intrinsic value, in more depth.

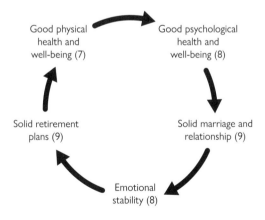

Figure 2.2 Current Inter-related Cycle of Priorities

As you can see, after 3 months of therapy based on the outcomes of the DTS-VADRA2016 and SAP there have been huge improvements in the five priority areas chosen by Mr Adams. He is making progress toward the set goals and, with 6 months to go before he retires, he is confident that he can achieve them. He continues to visit the weekly diabetes clinic but his fasting blood glucose numbers have ranged between 70 mg/dl and 90 mg/dl during each visit (this falls well below levels that determine evidence of diabetes). As he still has over 60 lb (27.22 kg) to lose, Mr Adams scored physical health and well-being a 7, and with four more therapy sessions yet to be had, his score of 8 for psychological health and well-being aims to be a 10, along with emotional stability, which is being addressed during sessions.

This case study highlights how the DTS-VADRA2016 has a valuable role to play in helping people identify and reduce their risks of developing an NCD, increasing overall health and well-being and ensuring a workable SAP is developed. It is imperative that goals set are both realistic and achievable, that the client is motivated to change and that tangible rewards are written into the plan. Mr Adams' reward was a 175 ml glass of cabernet sauvignon with his evening meal three times a week. This equates to approximately 9 units of alcohol in total. It is suggested through much research that red wine contains resveratrol, an antioxidant that appears to be healthy for the heart. One such study published in *Science Daily* in September 2006 stated that cabernet sauvignon red wine reduces the risk of NCD due to Alzheimer's type. This work was led by Dr Jun Wang at the Mount Sinai School of Medicine (Wang et al. 2006).

Chapter 3

The Use of Hypnotherapy with People Living with Dementia

In 2002, I was working at Highfield Care in the UK as their dementia specialist. It was at a time when things within the dementia care home sector needed to change. It was also a time when I wanted to change the way in which therapy was both viewed and provided to people living with any form of NCD. My motivation was to drive forward those changes, therefore I needed to find something that could improve the quality of life of people experiencing their unique journey of cognitive change. At that time, we did have a few new cognitive enhancers (acetylcholinesterase inhibitors) such as Aricept (donepezil) and Exelon (rivastigmine), which had been approved to be marketed in the UK in 1997. However, in my clinical experience we were seeing a high volume of antipsychotic (neuroleptic) medicines being prescribed to "manage" the behavioral and psychological symptoms of dementia (BPSD). Of course, these medicines are prescribed off-license as they are not approved to treat such symptoms of dementia.

Later, in 2008, alongside esteemed colleagues such as Dr Graham Stokes, Professor Clive Ballard and others, I was part of the All Party Political Group on Dementia (APPG) who held an inquiry at Westminster into the prescription of antipsychotic drugs to people with dementia living in care homes. The result of this was a report called "Always a Last Resort," whose aim is to ensure such medicine is prescribed only after all other options have been exhausted (APPG 2008). At that time I was the senior dementia consultant at Southern Cross Healthcare and informed the inquiry about my clinical experiences. However, back in 2002, overprescribing of these medicines was commonplace, and from the 2008 inquiry, it became evident that use of these drugs was leading to premature (and therefore unavoidable) mortality of patients living with an NCD who were being prescribed them.

I knew there had to be other ways of supporting people as they trudged down the most challenging paths of their journey; I just had to find it. After searching, researching and following up on various forms of non-pharmacological therapies, or talking therapies, ranging from counseling to Gestalt, I happened to learn about how hypnotherapy was beneficial in helping people overcome many psychological traumas, habits and addictions. After much thought I decided to embark on a diploma course in Liverpool to train as a hypno-psychotherapist, with the aim of using such techniques with my patients who had an NCD diagnosis. I was accepted as a student by the National College of Hypnosis and Psychotherapy and commenced my initial training in 2003. By 2005, I had my Diploma in Hypnosis and Hypnotherapy and Psychology and Psychotherapy, and a new friend, Dr Simon Duff, who was to become my co-researcher on the use of hypnotherapy in this very complex field, and who is now one of my closest friends and confidantes. We had both decided to proceed with our training in order to gain our Advanced Diploma in Hypno-Psychotherapy, and for that we needed to conduct a piece of primary research.

Dr Simon Duff is an accomplished forensic psychologist and currently Deputy Director of Forensic Programmes at the Faculty of Medicine and Health Sciences within the

University of Nottingham. His clinical work is based at the Merseycare NHS Trust Community Service, Mersey Forensic Psychology Service and The Scott Clinic. At the time we embarked on our research back in 2003, he was at the University of Liverpool.

Why I Chose This Research Project

On the very first day of my training I put two questions to the lecturer. First, I asked him whether hypnotherapy could be used with people who had a diagnosis of dementia. He responded that he did not know. Second, I asked whether it could be used with those who had severe hearing impairments and those who were regarded as legally deaf. Again, he responded that he did not know. The answers given were what I anticipated, so I do not mean to be discourteous to the lecturer, for whom I have the utmost respect. From that moment on, my intention was to discover, through primary research, whether hypnosis could work in some positive way for my patient group.

The Research

During a literature search, we came across some evidence that suggested there could be some benefits to this intervention. In 2001, Simon and Canonico reported that hypnosis had been used successfully in reducing the anxiety of a patient requiring lumbar punctures (Simon and Canonico 2001). That same individual was a needle phobe and was living with an NCD. This contradicted the belief of Spiegal and Spiegal, who, in 1978, stated that the ability to concentrate and attend for a sustained period of time is necessary for hypnosis to have positive outcomes (Spiegal and Spiegal 1978). This would mean that individuals with deficits in such areas would not be suitable for this type of therapy. Further evidence that suggested that the use of hypnosis and hypnotherapy could be beneficial was provided by Welden and Yesavage in 1982. In this case, 24 matched pairs of patients with dementia attended either a relaxation training group or a current affairs discussion group for 1 hour three times a week over a 3-month period. Instructions within the relaxation group included progressive muscle relaxation and a self-hypnosis technique. Those who learned self-hypnosis showed improvement on ratings of behavioral function compared with the control group, and additionally just over 40 percent were no longer in need of hypnotic medicines. However, no member of the control group was able to discontinue such medicines.

It was apparent that evidence gleamed from published literature indicated that hypnosis and hypnotherapy can impact positively on quality of life for people experiencing their journey through NCDs. This was encouraging and thus the research proposal was compiled and submitted to the appropriate ethics committee. The aim of the research was to determine whether this approach could positively influence quality of life and thus play a part in true person centered care approaches, therapies, interventions and techniques. As Professor Tom Kitwood stated in 1997, "dementia care involves empowering individuals and promoting interpersonal relationships" (Kitwood 1997). This therapy, if proven to demonstrate positive clinical outcomes, would be one of the ways in which this could be achieved.

The initial research project included active participants who received hypnotherapy once a week for 9 months, a control group and a neutral group. Outcomes were so positive that we followed up with a longitudinal study 12 months post completion of the initial research. Again, we saw some surprising results. I do not want to spend this entire chapter talking about the research, which was published in three peer-reviewed clinical journals and can be found here:

- Duff, S.C. and Nightingale, D.J. (2005) "The efficacy of hypnosis in changing the quality of life in patients with dementia. A pilot-study evaluation." *European Journal of Clinical Hypnosis,* 6(2), 20–29.

- Duff, S.C. and Nightingale, D.J. (2006) "Long term outcomes of hypnosis in changing the quality of life in patients with dementia." *European Journal of Clinical Hypnosis,* 7(1), 2–8.

- Duff, S.C. and Nightingale, D.J. (2007) "Alternative approaches to supporting people with dementia: Enhancing quality of life through hypnosis." *Alzheimer's Care Today,* 8(4), 321–331.

However, the seven key areas that were found to have a positive impact for those receiving hypnotherapy as measured against those who did not, can be seen in Figures 3.1 to 3.7. They show data over a 9-month period and at 21 months for each of the three groups. Figure 3.8 demonstrates the mean change in overall quality of life.

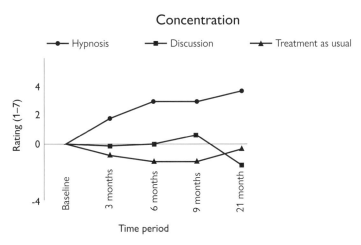

Figure 3.1 Concentration, over a 9-month period and at 21 months for the hypnosis group (HG), discussion group (DG) and treatment-as-usual group (TG)

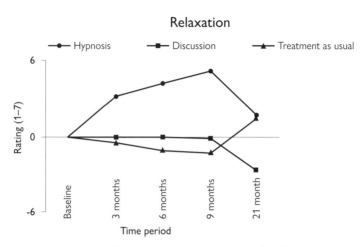

Figure 3.2 Relaxation, over a 9-month period and at 21 months for the hypnosis group (HG), discussion group (DG) and treatment-as-usual group (TG)

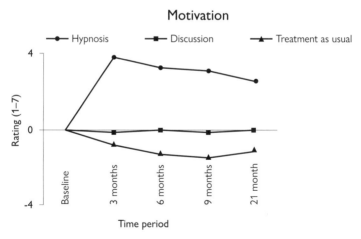

Figure 3.3 Motivation, over a 9-month period and at 21 months for the hypnosis group (HG), discussion group (DG) and treatment-as-usual group (TG)

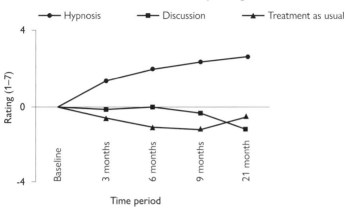

Figure 3.4 Activities of daily living, over a 9-month period and at 21 months for the hypnosis group (HG), discussion group (DG) and treatment-as-usual group (TG)

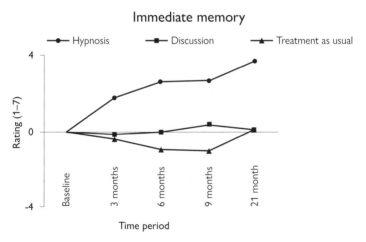

Figure 3.5 Immediate memory, over a 9-month period and at 21 months for the hypnosis group (HG), discussion group (DG) and treatment-as-usual group (TG)

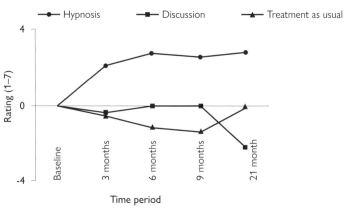

Figure 3.6 Memory for significant events, over a 9-month period and at 21 months for the hypnosis group (HG), discussion group (DG) and treatment-as-usual group (TG)

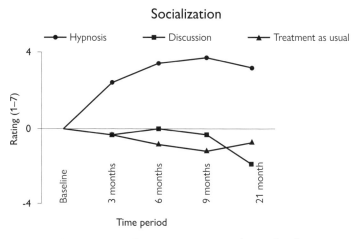

Figure 3.7 Socialization, over a 9-month period and at 21 months for the hypnosis group (HG), discussion group (DG) and treatment-as-usual group (TG)

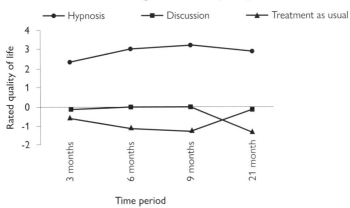

Figure 3.8 Mean change in overall quality of life, over a
9-month period and at 21 months for the hypnosis group (HG),
discussion group (DG) and treatment-as-usual group (TG)

As you can see, hypnosis has much to offer. I will provide two hypotheses as to why this therapy works. First, people with NCDs often find themselves living in a world where thinking is negative; where images and belief systems are pessimistic at best. For example, looking at someone who is struggling to remember a name, a face or an object, if we are able to take the person into a deep state of relaxation and replace negative thoughts, images and belief systems with positive ones, then it makes sense there will be improvements in various cognitive functions. Second, we know that at some point people will have difficulty with their sleep patterns. This is due to damage to the reticular activating system (RAS), which is a diffuse network of nerve pathways in the brainstem connecting the spinal cord, cerebrum and cerebellum, and mediating the overall level of consciousness. In other words, it is similar to a light switch in that it switches on and off conscious awareness. We know that people with NCD due to Alzheimer's disease have a much lower production of the neurochemical acetylcholine.

This chemical functions as a neurotransmitter sending signals from one brain cell to another. It causes muscles to contract, activates pain responses and regulates endocrine and rapid eye movement (REM) sleep functions. Are we actively stimulating production of acetylcholine when we induce hypnosis? During the induction stage the body becomes more and more relaxed, allowing the brain to go through various brain wave states. When the person is in deep hypnosis the brain shows a delta wave pattern associated with deep, dreamless sleep. Perhaps that deep, healing and cathartic state of relaxation is providing the sleep that cannot be achieved in the normal state due to dysfunction of the RAS. This could explain why, 12 months post therapy, some active participants continued to have positive benefits.

Following publication of the research (Duff and Nightingale 2005, 2006, 2007), I developed a training program for clinical hypnotherapists in order for them to provide this therapy to people living with an NCD. To date, I have taught over 300 clinicians, including medical doctors, psychologists and psychotherapists to use this approach.

The following case study details a case where hypnotherapy was used, how it was used and the positive outcomes that were achieved from it. The patient's name and place of residence have been changed for the sake of patient confidentiality and anonymity.

CASE STUDY

The medical definition of hypnosis is that it is a trance-like state of altered conscious awareness that resembles sleep but is induced by a person whose suggestions are readily accepted by the patient. It goes on to define hypnotherapy as a form of psychotherapy that facilitates suggestion, reduction or analysis by means of hypnosis.

Helen was 73 years of age with a diagnosis of NCD due to Alzheimer's disease. Additionally, she had chronic and severe arthritis that did not appear to be responding to medication. She had lived in Park Stanton Nursing Home for almost 3 years and had two very supportive daughters. Her husband, Billy, had passed away due to asbestosis a little over 12 months before I received the referral from her GP. Helen was having difficulty with pain management, relaxing, sleeping and remembering her two daughters. When assessing patients who live in a nursing home, or those who require full-time nursing care, I use Reisberg's Global Deterioration Scale (GDS) (Reisberg et al. 1982) to ascertain where they are in terms of their neurocognition. The MMSE or other screening tools are of little use in establishing whether a person at this stage of their journey is suitable for hypnotherapy. In the case of Helen, her score was 4, which equates to moderate cognitive decline (see Table 3.1).

Table 3.1 Reisberg's Global Deterioration Scale (GDS)

Diagnosis	Stage	Signs and symptoms
No dementia	**Stage 1: No cognitive decline**	In this stage the person functions normally, has no memory loss and is mentally healthy. People with *no* dementia would be considered to be in Stage 1
No dementia	**Stage 2: Very mild cognitive decline**	This stage is used to describe normal forgetfulness associated with aging; for example, forgetfulness of names and where familiar objects have been left. Symptoms are not evident to loved ones or the physician
No dementia	**Stage 3: Mild cognitive decline**	This stage includes increased forgetfulness, slight difficulty concentrating, decreased work performance. People may get lost more often or have difficulty finding the right words. At this stage, a person's loved ones will begin to notice a cognitive decline. Average duration: 7 years before onset of dementia

cont.

Diagnosis	Stage	Signs and symptoms
Early-stage	Stage 4: Moderate cognitive decline	This stage includes difficulty concentrating, decreased memory of recent events and difficulties managing finances or traveling alone to new locations. People have trouble completing complex tasks efficiently or accurately and may be in denial about their symptoms. They may also start withdrawing from family or friends, because socialization becomes difficult. At this stage a physician can detect clear cognitive problems during a patient interview and exam. Average duration: 2 years
Mid-stage	Stage 5: Moderately severe cognitive decline	People in this stage have major memory deficiencies and need some assistance to complete their daily activities (dressing, bathing, preparing meals). Memory loss is more prominent and may include major relevant aspects of current lives; for example, people may not remember their address or phone number and may not know the time or day or where they are. Average duration: 1.5 years
Mid-stage	Stage 6: Severe cognitive decline (middle dementia)	People in Stage 6 require extensive assistance to carry out daily activities. They start to forget names of close family members and have little memory of recent events. Many people can remember only some details of earlier life. They also have difficulty counting down from ten and finishing tasks. Incontinence (loss of bladder or bowel control) is a problem in this stage. Ability to speak declines. Personality changes, such as delusions (believing something to be true that is not), compulsions (repeating a simple behavior, such as cleaning), or anxiety and agitation may occur. Average duration: 2.5 years
Late-stage	Stage 7: Very severe cognitive decline (late dementia)	People in this stage have essentially no ability to speak or communicate. They require assistance with most activities (e.g. using the toilet, eating). They often lose psychomotor skills, for example, the ability to walk. Average duration: 2.5 years

From research we ascertained that a score of 1–4 results in the best outcomes from hypnotherapy. However, in clinical practice, we will always carry out an appropriate pre-hypnotherapy assessment prior to making a decision regarding suitability. I have had successful results with those who fall into 5 and even 6 of Reisberg's criteria.

Helen's score of 4 and her ability to express her thoughts and feelings about joint pain, the inability to relax or sleep without intermittent waking and not recognizing the faces of her two daughters was enough for me to consider the use of hypnotherapy. In this case, I assessed Helen as having the ability to consent to hypnotherapy as she was able to understand what would happen and retain that information long enough to repeat it back to me. In addition, and in this case, her GP and daughters also agreed that hypnosis would be an appropriate therapy. In cases where consent cannot be obtained, assent may be accepted as long as the therapy being administered is in the best interests of the patient.

I learned that Helen was a very visual person, so my test for suitability for her to receive hypnosis was based on the following visual exercise:

> Helen. Please close your eyes and be guided by my voice. You are walking through the shopping center when you see a little girl. She is smiling and carrying a balloon. She wears a beautiful dress. You smile at her and continue on your way. Please open your eyes Helen.

She was able to close and open her eyes as instructed. In addition, when I asked her the color of the balloon she said yellow and the dress was pink. This indicated to me that therapy based on guided visual imagery (GVI) was the most appropriate.

My approach to clinical hypnotherapy has six key stages, which are made up of the following:

1. Eye closure (induction stage).

2. Progressive muscle relaxation (induction stage).

3. Trigger word (induction stage).

4. Deepener (hypnosis stage).

5. Ideo motor response or ideo sensory response and therapy (hypnotherapy stage).

6. Termination (bringing the person back to conscious awareness).

I will discuss each of these stages as we work through Helen's session, and the inclusion of self-hypnosis, which I teach for both the conscious and unconscious state.

Self-hypnosis

Self-hypnosis, which is a form of self-relaxation, is a breathing technique that I teach to patients who have an NCD in order for them to use between weekly hypnotherapy sessions. Wherever possible, I also teach this to the main caregiver so they can enable and support my patient to use the technique each and every day. I taught Helen's daughter Karen so she could encourage and support her mother. I established Helen's favorite place – a place she prefers to be more than anywhere else in the world. For her it is sitting on the edge of Lake Coniston, Cumbria, on a warm summer's day. This favorite place is her safe, special place throughout hypnotherapy and self-relaxation sessions.

The process will be different for different patients, so for Helen the process, which I always record for the patient, was as follows:

Helen. I will see you each week but each day, I would like you to do this following exercise with your daughter Karen. As you are sitting comfortably in your chair, I want you to close your eyes and take a nice deep breath. As you breathe out I want you to feel the tension, stress and pain leave your body. That's good. Breathe in – and out. Relaxing, relaxing. Breathe in – and out. Sinking deeper and deeper into the chair. Breathe in – and out. Relaxing more and more and going to your special place. Breathe in one more time – and out.

You're now in your special place. Stay there and relax for as long as your body needs to relax. That's good Helen.

When patients do this daily, it becomes easier and easier and the benefit is that it supplements weekly hypnotherapy sessions and makes the induction process of hypnosis much quicker and easier for the patient.

Eye closure

Eye closure is a relatively straightforward part of the process where I ask Helen to focus on a point on the ceiling. I ask her not to blink. As she does this, I make suggestions that the muscles at the backs of her eyes are getting tired and that at any time she can simply relax and close her eyes.

Progressive muscle relaxation

At this point, I ask Helen to focus on her breathing and allow my voice to be her guide. Just to listen to my voice and relax. I suggest that each muscle in her body, each sinew, relaxes and that with each word I speak and each breath she takes, she sinks deeper and deeper into relaxation. More comfortable; the pain and discomfort melting away. I do this from the top of her head to the tips of her toes, making the appropriate and necessary suggestions as her body posture and facial expressions change, indicating a deep state of relaxation has been reached.

Trigger word

The trigger word is used as follows: "Helen. In a few moments' time I'm going to say the word 'now' and when I say the word 'now' in a few moments' time it will be a sign for you to relax as deeply as you wish to relax today. So, ready, 'now.'" Helen's facial expression becomes more peaceful and less tense and her breathing becomes much more relaxed. At this stage I am encouraged that she is entering the hypnogogic phase.

Deepener

The deepener is when I count her down from ten to one. As I count her down from ten to one she leaves her room and makes her way down to Coniston Lake, her safe place. On the count of one I suggest she steps into her safe place – a place where no one and nothing can go without her permission. There is no pain or discomfort in her special place. There are no problems with her memory in her special place. Whenever she is there, she is relaxed and in control. I suggest that she can see, hear, smell, touch and taste things with much more clarity and positive meaning. I ask her to enjoy the moment: the gentle breeze, the blue sky and singing birds, he warmth from the sun. After a pause of 2 minutes, I ask Helen to sit next to the water.

At this juncture, my job is to access her unconscious mind, which is hiding behind a sliding door. I must open that door by asking permission to speak with her unconscious mind and resolve the current challenges being faced by Helen. Once that door opens, and access is granted, the critical factor, or hidden observer, is ensuring I remain both professional and ethical and that I don't lead Helen into something that is uncomfortable or unpleasant and not ready to be addressed. Should I do that, the critical factor will close the door on me. It is the part of the conscious mind that allows or blocks information from the unconscious mind. I do this by asking for a sign from a part of her body – the IMR. The process I used resulted in the little finger on her left hand rising into the air. That was permission granted. That finger was asked to stay where it was and to lower at any time Helen was feeling uncomfortable and did not wish to proceed. This did not happen.

For any clinical or medical hypnotherapists reading this chapter, it has been my experience that the IMR elicited from people living with an NCD is much more pronounced – even if the patient has severe immediate memory dysfunction.

As I have accessed Helen's unconscious mind, I now proceed with the therapy. In this session, I use GVI to help her let go of certain negative images and experiences, including pain and discomfort, the fuzziness and the cloud that are making her forget the faces of her daughters (this disorder is relatively common in NCDs and is referred to as prosopagnosia). I make the suggestion that she can put all these things in an empty basket that is anchored to the ground. Many, many balloons are attached to the basket, which is big or small, depending on how much it is to be filled. Helen has 2 minutes to disconnect from those negative images and experiences by placing them in the basket. Once done, I ask that she release the basket and watch as it drifts high into the sky, eventually disappearing into a solitary cloud, taking away all that it contains within it.

Termination

Termination is when I ask Helen's little finger to fall in line with the rest of the fingers on both hands and allow the conscious mind to take control of all fingers and thumbs on both hands. I then reinforce the self-hypnosis technique before counting up from one to ten and bringing Helen back into her room; back into the present.

The positive outcomes for Helen have been clear for all to see. Her pain is managed to an extent that she has more physical freedom and she can both relax and sleep much better. Owing to constantly reinforcing, in hypnosis, and with the use of the spaced retrieval technique, again in hypnosis, Helen is now able to recognize both her daughters. (The spaced retrieval technique is a technique requiring the patient to rehearse certain information to be learned (and remembered) at increasing spaced intervals. For example, the clinician would say "My name is Dr Dan. What is my name?" The patient would reply immediately. The clinician would then say "My name is Dr Dan," then pause for 5 seconds before asking "What is my name?") Weekly sessions of hypnotherapy are ongoing at the time of writing.

From research and clinical experience, the clinician can expect to see improvements by week 4, though typically six sessions are planned following the initial consult.

Clinicians must understand that there is a huge difference between using hypnotherapy with this cohort and using it with those wishing to lose weight or cease smoking. For example, it is essential that the clinician have a full understanding of NCDs, disease pathology and how it impacts individually on the person. Another key difference is the time it takes to complete the induction phase and take the person into a deep state of relaxation. The clinician can spend up to an hour on this part of the process alone. Yet another key difference is the length of time it may take to establish a therapeutic alliance. The first two meetings are likely to be spent on exercises based around getting to know each other and building a relationship founded on warmth, honesty, genuineness and transparency.

Suggested Use by Non-Trained Clinicians and Carers

Schedule 20 minutes for this session, which should be carried out in a quiet, comfortable place where there will be no disturbances. Talk in a slow, calm voice. Encourage the person to select a positive affirmation, such as "I am focused and able to concentrate."

Ask the person to close their eyes and take five deep breaths. Ask them to imagine that all of the tension is draining out of their body. Now ask the person to imagine a sunset; describe to them all the colors and suggest that they watch as the sun sinks below the horizon and the evening stars begin to come out. Now, tell them:

> Relax each area at a time as you move up through your body. Become aware of your feet and relax that area. Now bring your awareness up through your ankles, knees, thighs, hips, stomach, chest, shoulders, neck and up into

your head behind your eyes, and then to a point above the top of your head.

Count down from ten to one and say:

> You are now in a deep state of relaxation. You are letting all the negativity, such as negative emotions, experiences and images, drift away.

Repeat this process a number of times before slowly counting up from one to ten and orienting the person back to the present moment.

Technique to Use During Limited Time Consults

The average consultation time for a GP is approximately 10 minutes. There is a great deal to be achieved within that 10-minute window, so what technique based on hypnotherapy can be done in such a short space of time?

Laughter increases production of antibodies and releases endorphins, the body's natural painkillers. To help a patient leave the consulting room in a happier, more positive state than when they entered, the following 2-minute therapy can be used:

> Close your eyes and take five deep breaths with me. Excellent. Now, relax your head, shoulders and arms, and let your chin rest on your chest. Good. Now, create an image in your mind that makes you feel happy. That's right, now focus on that image and really feel how happy it makes you. So happy in fact that you smile on the inside, which makes you smile on the outside. Excellent. You're already feeling so much better. Now, open your eyes. Look at me. Let's laugh. Let's laugh together. There, isn't that better?

If this is done at the beginning of the consult, the patient will be in a much more positive and relaxed mindset. The patient will also be more accessible for examinations, palpations and discussions around diagnostics and treatment suggestions.

Hypnotherapy has been shown, through empirical research and clinical practice, to improve the quality of life of people with various types of NCDs. Whether the person lives in their family home or a nursing home, assisted living community, memory care community or other care environment, similar improvements can be achieved.

Chapter 4

The Nightingale Model of Enriched Care

When I first entered the very challenging arena of dementia care as a charge nurse back in 1992, my colleagues went to great pains to educate me in how *not to care* for people living with NCDs.

I entered this field of care after spending time in forensic learning disability services and there I witnessed draconian practices that wouldn't have been out of place in some of the institutional museums that existed during the days of Alois Alzheimer.

First, there was an expectation that everyone would be up and dressed after having breakfast and sitting in the lounge (*sorry – day room!*) in time for the day staff to come on duty. Likewise, everyone would be in bed in time for the night staff to take over.

Second, nobody ever went out! The mere mention of Fred being supported to go to the pub on a Friday night filled the care team with dread. (*I may as well have asked them to work for a month salary-free – I think the response would have been less frightful!*)

Third, and this was when I decided that I would make this field my area of expertise in order that I could actually begin to change things, there was constant abuse of the people living in a care home environment: sometimes subtle, sometimes blatant, but always detrimental to the physical and psychological health and well-being of the individual. There was no respect. There was no dignity. There was no choice. When I witnessed a lady of about 87 years of age being woken by a care worker and a nurse at 5.30am I was so angry that I felt tears welling up inside me – for they had a bowl of cold water and were flicking it into this lady's face. Their feet never touched the ground!

It was obvious that this place, like many others, was being run for the convenience of those who worked there.

Thankfully, we have moved forward since then. However, have we moved forward enough? Fast enough? In a way that truly demonstrates to people living with an NCD, their loved ones, employed caregivers, friends and, yes, even professionals, that it is a unique journey for each person? That medicine is not the only intervention available? That by entering the world of the very people we are supporting, we can make a positive difference?

It has been many years since Professor Tom Kitwood and his colleagues first introduced the concept of person centered care to the medical and psychology professions. It might be useful at this juncture to identify the key features of what I refer to as true person centered care.

- True person centered care accentuates the positive and minimizes the negative.

- True person centered care focuses on strengths and abilities rather than weaknesses and disabilities.

- True person centered care promotes well-being and minimizes ill-being – a positive rather than a negative approach.

- True person centered care focuses on the perspective of the individual, rather than that of the caregiver.

- True person centered care is planned around the individual and not the care home environment – not task orientated care.

- True person centered care sees behaviors that challenge others as an expression of feelings.

- True person centered care sees behaviors that challenge others as a means of communication – the onus is on the caregiver to interpret as far as possible.

- True person centered care acknowledges that there is always a reason for a behavior.

- True person centered care accepts the reality of the person and does not insist on bringing him or her into our reality, which can cause distress to the person; for example, not telling a person that their mother is dead when he or she calls for them.

- True person centered care acknowledges each person as a unique individual in all their words and actions.

- True person centered care does not use detracting words or labels, e.g. "uncooperative" or "a wanderer" or "a feeder" or "a sufferer."

- True person centered care is implemented by the caregivers, who try to see things through the person's eyes and not their own.

If you consider the key features as described above, there was no reason why Tom Kitwood's concept of person centered care was not being implemented in the care home environment immediately after he published his work – but it wasn't. None of this can be described as rocket science; all of it can be described as part of a humanitarian approach to enable a person to enjoy a quality of life based around their strengths, dignity, respect and choice, and all were strangely absent in a large bulk of the sector in 1992. This brings me to the question of why this was the case, and continues to be the case, in some establishments.

So why is it that many care homes still find it difficult to provide true person centered care to those living in such communities? Before I try to answer this question it may be useful to the reader if I clarify my own perception of *true person centered care*. To do this I will simply quote a gentleman who lives in a care home in Manchester, UK:

> I guess this term means all about me doesn't it?

Quite simply *yes it does*. The term "person centered care" has become diluted over the years because it has been so widely used.

It is the responsibility of each and every person to ensure that it once again becomes strengthened. We can do this by remembering that it is all about enabling a person to maintain their sense of well-being, sense of personhood, sense of identity and sense of self. True person centered care is about enabling an individual to *be*. It is not about *doing* things for people. It is about changing all our practices.

The Nightingale Model of Enriched Care can, and does, make it possible for caregivers, managers, directors, proprietors, commissioners and regulators to change their existing practices and make the shift from task orientated care to person centered care – all you need to do is accept that there are no rules in terms of interventions and approach and that whatever your own personal biases may be, they should never influence those interventions or approaches.

That said, there is a challenge far greater than those posed by people living with dementia, and that challenge comes from a number of external and internal sources. It is these sources that must subscribe to this model to ensure that we have total and complete consistency in approach and continuity of care – this will lead to a truly remarkable and positive lived experience for those who are on their journey through cognitive change, loved ones, caregivers and those members of the direct care teams who are the providers of care and who are enabling the journey. What's more, we will all agree with the care being delivered, there will be consistency in approach and continuity of care. There will be a structure we can all follow and a radical change in care concepts will be forced upon local and central government.

So who really needs to change?

1. *The government* – and it doesn't matter which political party hold the power. In England, "Living Well With Dementia – a national dementia strategy," was published in February 2009 (DoH 2009) and in February 2008 Westminster held an APPG inquiry on the use of antipsychotic drugs in residential care homes ("Always A Last Resort: Inquiry into the prescription of antipsychotic drugs to people with dementia living in care homes," APPG 2008). I was one of the witnesses at Westminster, along with eminent clinicians including Professor Clive Ballard and Dr Graham Stokes. The report was produced to inform the National Dementia Strategy. These two proactive parliamentary initiatives are indicative that central government in the UK is beginning to listen to the voices of people living with NCDs, their loved ones and caregivers, advocates and professionals. It has taken a long time for these voices to be heard and now it is down to the rest of us to maintain that momentum so that care remains a key focus at every level, not just in the UK, but in other developed countries too. This Model of Enriched Care can assist care providers in the implementation of their national strategies. Canada was the 30th country to implement their strategy in 2018.

2. *Regulatory bodies*, in particular the Care Quality Commission (CQC), departments of social services and health. These bodies must demonstrate a further understanding of the psychological impact term-inology can have on those living with NCDs. I refer in particular to terms such as Elderly Mentally Ill (EMI), unit and, even worse, an EMI unit. This terminology

can be regarded as a personal detraction, a term of abuse. After all, who wants to be labeled as being Elderly Mentally Ill? Who wants to be referred to as living in a unit? As we will all readily agree, people on this journey are not always elderly and none is mentally ill in the way modern society perceives mental illness, nor in the way that the International Statistical Classification of Diseases and Related Health Problems, 10th edition (ICD-10; WHO 2016) and DSM-5 diagnose mental illness. This means there is indeed a contradiction here, and one that we need to evaluate further. Though dementia is a neurodegenerative disorder, is it really a form of mental illness? I suggest that the answer is no, which is the rationale behind the recommendations in "Always a Last Resort" that antipsychotic medicines not be prescribed for the behavioral challenges symptomatic of NCDs. One could postulate that NCDs often lead to such things as hallucinations, neuroses and sometimes psychoses, but these illnesses may accompany any of the primary NCDs – they are not the disorder per se. Thus, we are moving away from the medical model and adopting a social, psycho-social and psychological approach to supporting people through the challenging aspects of their journey. Nor do people live in units. They live in houses, flats, apartments, homes. So, we appeal to everyone to drop the demeaning terminology, remove it from your minds completely and we will see a positive improvement in quality of life. This is because something as subtle as this changes one's own thoughts, ideologies and perceptions. Have we not done the same in the field of learning/intellectual disabilities? A strong partnership is needed among those who own and invest in care services, directors, managers, commissioners and regulators.

3. *Care home proprietors* and this includes the corporate, profit-making services as well as smaller operators, social services and voluntary services. If these services take on board the model described in this book and adopt it as a minimum standard, the following will be achieved: both the physical and psychological well-being of those living in such communities will be enhanced; the progression of cognitive decline will be radically reduced, thus increasing life span; and members of the direct care team will be motivated and feel supported during their very challenging but meaningful roles, thus reducing staff turnover and achieving a consistent team approach. In conclusion, you will be providing not only person centered care, but *true* person centered and person focused care. For example, one of the recommendations made for inclusion in the National Dementia Strategy in England is that dementia training should be mandatory for all those supporting people along their journey. By this, I am referring to quality training and not just a day or a couple of hours. Training needs to be ongoing and continuous, and should include understanding and implementation of *true* person centered and person focused care, communication skills and the risks and benefits of antipsychotic medicines. Presently, this level of training in many countries falls well short of an acceptable standard. Members of the direct care teams should receive a basic, underpinning knowledge of the various types of NCDs and the impact they have on those living with them and their loved ones before even meeting those requiring care and support. Resources must be made available in order for the model to have maximum impact. I have implemented this model within a number of care communities during my time as a clinical dementia

specialist, and the results have been outstanding – many examples of which are described in this book. If we are serious about making a positive change, then examples of best practice must be demonstrated by those people who lead services from the top down.

4. *Professionals*, including doctors, psychologists, psychotherapists, nurses and social workers in all disciplines and at all levels. Another of the recommendations made by the APPG inquiry mentioned earlier was that more emphasis should be placed on NCDs in the training curriculum for doctors, especially family practitioners, and that there needs to be improved education for them on behavioral and psychological symptoms, antipsychotic medicines and alternative solutions. Also, that care homes must receive effective support from family practitioners, mental health nurses, psychologists and psychiatrists, with the inclusion of regular, proactive visits. A better understanding of the positive impact of non-aversive interventions that draw on the use of psychotherapy, cognitive behavior therapy, hypno-psychotherapy and other psycho-social approaches and techniques would make a huge difference. However, there must also be adequate access to these services. Should psycho-social interventions be more readily available, then the need for chemical restraint would be significantly reduced. Also, if professionals foster and develop the following Model of Enriched Care, we will see care facility staff following their lead.

Collectively, there needs to be a massive change in beliefs, attitudes and current care service practices if we are to implement person centered and person focused care in its true sense.

The remainder of this chapter describes the Nightingale Model of Enriched Care and demonstrates how and why it has worked during my clinical practice and how other professionals can use it to enhance their practice and service delivery. So, whether you are living with dementia, are a loved one of someone with dementia, are a professional or student, a member of the direct care team, a director or manager, a proprietor, a commissioner or regulator of services, what follows is of value to you.

The Model

Figure 4.1 demonstrates the fundamental principles of enriching the lives of people living through their unique journey of cognitive change. Having Alzheimer's disease, vascular NCD, Lewy body, Pick's or any other primary disorder is as unique as a fingerprint and impacts each person on an individual basis. In Chapter 2 I talked about the need for Shared Action Planning where the individual is in the driver's seat. This model supports that type of approach.

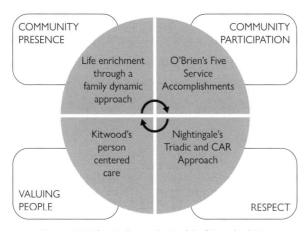

Figure 4.1 The Nightingale Model of Enriched Care

Figure 4.1 outlines the fundamental principles that underpin a truly enriched life for people living with cognitive change, their loved ones, friends and enablers. This model is relevant to people residing in care communities, and it is one I have developed following years of clinical experience in the field. This experience encompasses supporting not only the person in the driving seat, but their loved ones, carers, nurses and other professionals who are involved in the everyday lives of each individual faced by the many challenges this disability often brings. After all, it is a journey shared by all but experienced differently by each. It is their collective voices that have helped develop this model. There now follows a description of each component.

Life Enrichment Through a Family Dynamic Approach

The majority of people living together in a care community do so under unnatural conditions. Additionally, enablers are part of that core group. This means that in order to achieve the aim of this model, that is, to provide an enriched life, enablers must understand the complexities of family dynamics and group living. This includes issues ranging from similar interests and lifestyles, life experiences, personalities and characters to inner group conflict and problem solving. This model sees this as key to a successful living environment built on mutual understanding, respect and trust.

When thinking about family dynamics, it may be useful to think of them in two ways:

1. Positive family dynamics (PFD).

2. Negative family dynamics (NFD).

Here is an example of each:

- *PFD*: Tanya is very close to all members of her family. All members of that family are close to each other.

They enjoy family gatherings regularly and enjoy family holidays. If any of them need support in any way, they are always there for each other. Nobody ever enjoys life on their own, it is all shared. Nobody ever endures negative aspects of life on their own, it is all shared. None of Tanya's brothers, sisters, parents, aunts, uncles, nieces or nephews ever feels alone.

- *NFD*: Steve has not spoken to his father in about 10 years now and will never do so again. He is close to his mother, who recently remarried. However, he cannot be around her for too long as she is hyperactive. He has four older brothers but none of them are really close and none of them speak to their father. Steve forever asks himself: "If we really needed each other, would we be there?"

Now, just spend a few moments thinking about how your family dynamics impact on your thoughts, attitude and general behavior at any given time. You might like to jot those things down.

Now consider how family dynamics might be important to the people living in a care community. Each individual brings with them a family history, a background. Even if all those around the individual are now deceased, they still had a place within a family, however large or small. For those people who still have family around them, the dynamics change when one or more enter a care environment. Key to this are:

- A husband/wife relationship changes in a number of ways. Importantly, they are no longer living together on a full-time basis. This can lead to high levels of stress and anxiety on the part of both individuals. As members of the direct care and management team, you are now part of those dynamics. You must be able to empathize with the experiences each one is living.

You are able to do this by considering your own past or present situation. Ask yourself: "How would I feel if this happened to me?" Some people are relieved not to have the carer responsibility any longer. Others may feel an overwhelming sense of guilt. A husband, wife or life partner may want to spend every waking hour with their loved one, while another may not even be able to visit as the psychological pain of doing so is unbearable. For these reasons, and many more that are personal to each individual, the dynamics in this relationship change. The support you can give, first of all, is empathy, warmth and genuineness. Then look at ways and strategies by which you can facilitate a PFD between these two individuals, thus enhancing their quality of life as they recognize that you value their relationship needs – their need to be together, to have privacy and space, to be affectionate and intimate, to be loving and caring, to have misunderstandings, disagreements and arguments, to kiss and make up.

- A parent/child relationship changes in that very often that role is reversed. The child becomes the parent. To begin to explore this, just consider what might be happening here? Why does a son or daughter feel the need to take the role of decision maker? Let's look at what happens psychologically. We all feel disappointed by our childhood experiences with our parents to some extent: it just comes with being human. Some people were truly tortured by parents, the rest of us just got less than we wanted or imagine we needed and experienced some genuine deficits in some areas. Our parent, or parents, may have abused us in some way, or may just not have been as warm and nurturing as we would have hoped. Most of us arrive at adulthood with a longing and need to try to resolve any wounds by getting what we want/need from our actual parent and/or parent stand-ins (lovers, friends, bosses, etc.). And whether we feel good about our childhoods or not, we tend to see our parents as someone always around to take care of us. So when a parent becomes in need of care and support due to their age, illness or disease, or close to death, at least two things happen instantly. First, we realize we will never get from the parent what we didn't get as children; any last chance has now gone. We now fear that, with their death, we will be alone and unprotected in the world. Amanda, a 41-year-old family doctor, has regular nightmares about her mother's death and cries openly with fear at the thought of losing her. Emotionally, Amanda feels as though she is still a small child who genuinely would be unable to care for herself if her mother died. On one level, she has never adjusted to the fact that her mother will never nurture her to make up for her coldness when Amanda was young. On another level, she has not yet come to terms with the human condition – that we are all alone, finally, in the world. And from a spiritual perspective, Amanda has not resolved her spiritual beliefs in a way that she can see her own death as anything less than a tragedy.

If you find yourself faced with a situation where the child becomes the main carer, here are some suggestions that might help:

1. Try to discover the kind of relationship they had with each other prior to this role reversal. Was the relationship close or distant? Was there regular contact? Is there evidence of genuine love and compassion? Is the view of the child that he or she is expected to visit their mother or father – that it is just another task as part of a regular routine?

By establishing where people are within that relationship, you as a member of the direct care or management team can then decide the most appropriate way of supporting and enabling that relationship.

2. Establish a relationship with the son or daughter based on genuineness, empathy and warmth. A positive relationship here is more likely to encourage openness and transparency on their part. Find out if there is more than one son or daughter who is in a position to provide support to their parent and sibling. This reduces the likelihood of stress or anxiety in all concerned.

3. Recognize that the son or daughter will have a multitude of complex and seemingly contradictory feelings, and they are all normal. He or she will feel sad, angry, detached, frightened and panicked about their parent's situation, possibly grieved when they do die but also relieved. "Why relief?" you may ask. A sense of closure. It's all over. No more suffering for either party. It is possible that the son or daughter has been experiencing a living bereavement for a parent lost. This may explain the rollercoaster of emotions as mentioned above. Your role is to continue to support the relative for as long as necessary. As you have played a very important part in these dynamics, you too have the right to grieve and seek support from within the whole family concept.

4. Encourage members of the family to join support groups when appropriate. Helen found a support group for people whose family members had Alzheimer's disease. The group helped a lot, and she found she was not alone in having a life partner living through this journey.

Strange as it sounds, the experience of having a dying or ill parent is an opportunity more than it is a tragedy. The Buddhists believe that one cannot fully appreciate life until one has experienced and grasped the meaning of death. If you use this experience for growth, you may find that you become mature and self-reliant as never before, that you give up your myths about needing a perfect parent yourself, and that you have a heightened sense of the preciousness of life and a new set of priorities for yourself. Our parents are, after all, nothing more than imperfect beings who gave us a start in life but then have little real relevance to how we live that life. Their passing is perhaps sad but merely part of the way of things. For those with a strong spiritual sense, their passing is only a passing of the body, and we realize we can retain what is good about their gift of life for as long as we need.

If, as part of a dedicated and committed care team enabling people to live positively through their journey of dementia, you practice within the framework of this family dynamic concept, the remainder of this model will fit together like a jigsaw puzzle.

O'Brien's Five Service Accomplishments

These are often referred to as O'Brien's Five Accomplishments (or Five As) and are made up of:

1.   Community presence (see page 74).

2.   Community participation (see page 75).

3.   Competence.

4.   Relationships outside the context of a family.

5.   Choice.

The five As underpinned the Community Care Act in the early 1990s and were used to help develop services for people with learning/intellectual disabilities. This is a successful model that is of great significance and importance in terms of successful and active community living (O'Brien 1989). We will now look at these and consider their relevance as part of this model.

Community Presence

This relates to how care communities can have a *dominant* and *active* presence in the community. Other members of society may well know that there is a care home locally, but that is usually as much as they know – as much as they want to know! People with NCDs have been on the periphery of society for many, many years. Not any more – not if this model is adopted and implemented in the care home, which *must* be seen as part of the local community, not separate from it. How might you achieve this while protecting those who may be some of the most vulnerable members of society?

Many services organize summer fetes and other social events and, though this is often for the purposes of marketing, it is an ideal opportunity to encourage members of the mainstream community into the home, thus laying down the opportunity for new friendships to develop. These initiatives must be built upon and the service made transparent to outsiders in order to dispel the myth that the majority of care and nursing facilities are bad places to be.

Just think for a few moments about why the majority of people never plan to spend their last few years of life in a care home. Why do people believe such places ought to be avoided like the plague?

I'm sure you have been able to identify a number of reasons, but two key ones lie at the doors of the media, local and central government. The two factors I refer to are negative press from the media and a total and complete lack of government funding for essential elements such as staff training and development. I point this out because neither the press nor government agencies promote care homes in a good positive light: yes, extra care is very much on the agenda and definitely the future; however, during this lengthy transition, current care homes cannot just be ignored and left unsupported. Government agencies must help by investing both financially and through leadership with an agenda which includes proactive measures that will integrate every care service into the local community in the same way as has been achieved in the learning disability sector.

Community Participation

This relates to how people living in a care service can continue to participate in mainstream society and the local community. It goes side by side with community presence and enhances well-being by ensuring people maintain a *role* in life.

A care service that really focuses on *community participation* will utilize its resources to enable people to form and maintain the variety of ties, connections and relationships that constitute community life. Many of those people will know and be known by other members of the community, such as their next door neighbors and past co-workers. They will have acquaintances that they would regularly get in contact with to share an interest, and be members of community groups and associations will have participated in civic, cultural, and political life.

How can you, as a clinician, enable these activities and links to be maintained?

What other initiatives can you implement to ensure that full and complete community participation continues when an individual moves in to a care home?

Valuing People

Words (statements that make use of them) such as value, choice, dignity, respect and person centered have become diluted over the years. Here we explore why this has happened and how we can strengthen those concepts once again through adopting appropriate terminology and demonstrating their true meaning.

A care service that really focuses on *encouraging valued social roles* will utilize its resources to enable people to enjoy the dignity and status associated with positively regarded activities. It is vital that valued social roles are maintained for each and every one of us. It helps shape who we are as people, how we behave and are regarded in society. For example, Peter wakes up at 4am to get ready for an early shift at work. As an ex-police officer he would start work at 6am. How will you respond to Peter?

There are three options available.

First, you could tell him he no longer works as a police officer, that he retired many years ago and that he should go back to bed. Likely outcome? Agitation due to the fact his reality is different to yours.

Second, you could lie to him by telling him that today is his day off. Likely outcome? Agitation due to confusion over his shift patterns.

Third, you could engage him positively, acknowledging that he needs to get to work and entering his reality. You can then sit and have breakfast and a chat about his role in the force and gradually move away to a different subject and positive activity. Likely outcome? A sense of well-being for Peter due to your positive interaction with him.

For many years, there has been a national debate among professionals in the field about the ethics and dilemmas of such validation and acknowledgment. In conclusion, we all agree that the appropriate intervention is individual. That is to say, the example above was appropriate for Peter but one of the other interventions described may have a positive outcome for someone else.

It is not possible to stress enough that a valued social role has a huge positive impact on an individual living with dementia. So, whenever and wherever possible, ensure that you empower people to enjoy a valued role.

Respect

A care service that really focuses on *the true meaning of respect* will utilize its resources to enable people to receive the same level of respect as would be afforded any member of society.

Services must take responsibility to strive to enhance the reputation of people and present them in a positive light to others, so that they are still viewed as continuing to have a valued role in the community within which they live, that is, the care home, but also within society as a whole. This will lead to each individual being seen as a person as opposed to somebody with a memory problem, and strengthens the valued social role they will have.

Choice

A care service focusing on *promoting choice* will utilize its resources to enable people to increase control over their own lives. The England and Wales Mental Capacity Act 2005 is a powerful tool that is aimed at protecting those with a cognitive impairment. It tells us that we must do everything possible to support that individual to make their own decisions, and only when we are confident that somebody else needs to make a particular decision after exploring every possible avenue, must we do so in the best interests of that individual.

However, there is no doubt that we have a challenge with the issue of choice. It isn't always as simple as asking a person whether they would like a cup of tea or a cup of coffee. Why is this? One of the main things we need to make a choice is our imagination.

Just stop for a second and consider this: would you like to go to see a football game tonight or would you rather go out for dinner? Now think about what just happened. How did you make your choice? What happened in your mind that helped you make that decision? Perhaps you had images of past experiences; memories of seeing a game of football either on television or at a stadium; memories of going out to dinner. So, not only is our imagination used but also our memory system.

Therefore, one of the things we need to consider is: *why on earth do we ask people with memory challenges today what they would like to do tomorrow?* The answer is strikingly obvious: management of the care service.

Instead, we need to be making use of every resource at hand to ensure we are able to present the person with an engaging activity at the present time. When we do ask what a person would like to do, show them a picture that shows their choice, such as a person sitting out in the sun. What matters to an individual living with an NCD is what is happening at the present time. What happened 5 minutes ago, or what is about to happen in 5 minutes' time, is totally irrelevant. This is inclusion. This is empowerment. Is this idealism or a realistic option with some thought and application? I shall leave you to decide.

Kitwood's Person Centered Care

No book about this topic would be complete without the inclusion of the late Professor Tom Kitwood's vision of person centered care (Kitwood 1997). After all, this is what leads to the avoidance of malignant social psychology. However, most mainstream services still fail to implement true person centered care, blaming lack of resources, both human and financial.

This does not have to be the case. Fostering and developing the correct attitude right from the start does achieve true person centered care, thus ensuring quality of life and well-being is continuous. The term "person centered care" has become part of everyday language. My worry is that because of this, its true meaning has become somewhat diluted. So what exactly is meant by person centered care? Although the exact term used varies, there is a general consensus that "person centered" or "quality" care is focused on the individual, that it promotes independence and autonomy as opposed to control and that it encourages people to choose from reliable, flexible services. It is about inclusion, not exclusion, and tends to be provided by enablers who remain grounded in their care role.

By this, I mean it becomes all too easy for support staff, and nurses, to see their role in a care service as a job, a task. When this happens, task orientated care practices dominate and true person centered care is not possible. Therefore, to avoid this type of malignant care, members of the direct care teams *must* also feel valued and supported by their line managers.

In discussing the Nightingale Triadic and CAR Approach below, we will see how we can achieve true person centered care in the care home environment within the parameters of the existing financial and human resources.

Nightingale's Triadic and CAR Approach

The Triadic Approach focuses on the environment; adequate and appropriate training; and continued development and psycho-social support strategies, systems, mechanisms and interventions. The CAR Approach focuses on communication, *a*ttitude and *r*esponse.

This combination ensures that enablers learn to be *wholly positive and totally non-aversive* in the way they perceive NCDs as a unique experience and thus provide *support* on an individual basis. Barriers are broken down until removed completely, thus dissolving the "*us and them*" phenomenon. As a result, this leads to empowerment of the person with NCD, who can then receive the support required, when required, at a time convenient to that person without the fear of institutional neurosis being an outcome of malignant care strategies. We will look at each one of these elements in turn.

Environment

This is a key element in determining how an individual behaves at any given time, day or night, in a care home setting. Here I refer to both the external and internal environment. For example, Inclusive Design for Getting Outdoors (I'DGO), a research consortium consisting of a core group of academic researchers who, together with a wide range of partners, constitute a virtual center of excellence focusing on design of outdoor environments to include older people and disabled people, state that the inaccessibility and difficulties presented by many outdoor environments are a major problem affecting older people at present. This is further aggravated by a lack of awareness about design features that could support independent activities and make a difference to the quality of their daily lives.

The impact of the internal environment is further strengthened by what lies outside. Think about the following for a moment or two: You have lived all your life as an active member of society. You have developed an acceptance of environmental cues. Your brain has formulated an ecological inventory of all the things that help you orientate yourself to time and place, all the things that help you get from A to B, all the things that give you aesthetic pleasure, all the things that allow a sense of well-being, of personhood. You have interacted and have been interacted with. There has been stimulation of the senses too.

What are these things?

Well, just take a look around you. What do you see? What can you hear? What can you smell? Reach out and touch the thing closest to you. How does it feel? What can you taste?

Your environment gives you a real purpose. It is a key factor in helping shape you as a person. So, imagine entering a care home and no longer seeing the post box at the end of the street or the pub down the road; no longer smelling the aroma of home cooking; no longer seeing your own front door; no longer taking the trip to the shops; no longer having local signs that tell you where you are, where you are going. Include in the mix the fact that you have some kind of cognitive dysfunction – maybe your immediate memory is impaired, or your vision. Perhaps you have some macular degeneration or cataracts. Then there is the visual challenge that we know many people experience: the loss of ability to recognize colors at the low end of the color spectrum. How might this affect you when first arriving at the care home?

Your response is likely to be based on two powerful emotions: fear and anxiety. The transitions that each person experiences are different. However, for many individuals fear of the unknown leads to severe general anxiety. When someone is confronted with such negative experiences they will use whatever resources they have at hand to express their feelings. For a person living in a care home, their expressions are likely to be labeled as *challenging behavior*.

What we must always remember is that our role is *not* to manage people. Our role *is* to enable, empower and support them to have an enriched life. So, when developing your clinical skills, it is crucial that you do so by entering the individual's reality.

The German author and poet Christian Morganstern famously wrote "Home is not where you live but where they understand you." No matter where one lives, at the family home, or in a care home, living well, living safely and living comfortably are crucial to a positive state of well-being. Whether you are thinking about the outdoor area or inside the home, think about the environmental cues we all need and introduce them to the area. For example, it is important to develop a community within a community. By this I mean turning a bedroom door into the person's front door so the room becomes their house. They then step outside of their house into a community that is both stimulating and interactive as opposed to a typical care home corridor. They might walk past a shop window, a pub, café or market place. There is appropriate signage in the size, shape and color that give people the maximum opportunity to recognize what the sign is and the direction they are heading and where they are. Remember, the reality of the person you are providing a service to may well be different to yours – you may be living in the present day, but that person may be reliving 1973. If the surroundings are familiar and recognizable, then the possibility of fear and anxiety is reduced immensely; thus, behaviors that are seen as a challenge to the service are dramatically reduced. For example, the provision of elevated lighting such as street lights not only helps a person with NCD to see where they are going, but also reduces their uncertainty and trepidation.

This can greatly reduce the risk of sundowner syndrome, a phenomenon noticed by many relatives and staff that describes a change, somewhere around 4pm, when the person becomes more confused, more disorientated, restless and muddled, thus leading to heightened emotional responses and agitation. Research conducted by a group of Dutch scientists clinically tested the effect that long exposure to bright light and melatonin has on the functioning of people living with an NCD. The authors of the paper claim that, on the whole, light treatment could have clinically beneficial effects. The ceiling lights, more than three times brighter than those used as a comparison, also reduced depression by 19 percent. Light attenuated cognitive deterioration by 0.9 points on the MMSE questionnaire (Riemersma-van der Lek et al. 2008).

This clearly demonstrates how an appropriate environment can influence a positive state of well-being by negating the risk of ill-being.

There is much anecdotal evidence too. Helen, the director of a care facility in Birmingham, fed back to me that:

> Since changing our environment through the introduction of a community within a community philosophy, the residents are much happier and calmer. They are experiencing new things every day and one lady, Elsa, can find her own little house now. We painted her door and made it look similar to the front door she had been used to for over 50 years. Before we did that, staff always had to go with her. The staff team are happier too. This is only one part of what we do, but it has proven to be a vital part of true person centered approach.

Jack told me:

> Clocks. I grew up surrounding by clocks. I have lots of them here. I have one on my door. I know that I need to go through it. There are more inside it and they make me smile.

I watched Margaret as she made her way from her house down the street, which had a hairdressing salon and shop front. The dining room had been made into a café with a 1970s theme. She went inside and sat at the table. Margaret looked at a picture on the wall and smiled. She then got up, left the café and continued her journey. Clearly, for her, the environment was having a huge positive impact.

It might sometimes seem bizarre to those who do not have a cognitive change. Some critics argue that we are creating a false environment; that we don't have these things in our own houses. I would respond by saying that it really doesn't matter. In the grand scheme of things, if Peter wants to walk and put paper or envelopes into a box time and time again, and if this gives him a sense of purpose, a role, a sense of achievement, then it is something to encourage, not deter. If you can turn a frown into a smile, the purpose behind this approach has been met.

Adequate and appropriate training and continued development

Is it not a frightening thought that somebody can get a job as a caregiver supporting people who have an NCD without any training or basic idea of how people live through their journey? Nearly every specialist in this field of care would argue that adequate and appropriate training is vital. It is essential for training to be sustained and continuous and leadership and supervision are critical components to ensuring that true person centered care is delivered at each and every interaction.

Here we have a huge challenge. The challenge is that we must fill the gap between what we have as knowledge in terms of how true person centered care positively impacts on people, their relatives and carers and actually delivering it in the care home environment. As I pointed out earlier, Kitwood's work has been known for many years but we continue to fail his vision. As a clinician, I see this failure day in and day out. I have already identified why this might be, so will suggest ways in which we can plug this identified gap.

First, outcomes from all credible research must be translated for non-academics. So much is kept in academic journals that when I refer to it for a specific reason I am very often met with blank faces. Research outcomes that directly affect care practices must be included in all training and development courses. Senior managers and educators have a duty to ensure this is the case.

It is a pointless exercise asking people to attend a classroom-based training course if there is no experiential opportunity to complement theoretical learning. Courses are being developed regularly but it is essential that whatever training is delivered we start by asking four fundamental questions:

1. Why is the training required?

2. What are you aiming to achieve through the provision of training?

3. Who will deliver the training and what are their qualifications for doing so?

4. Is senior management in support of the initiative and will the required resources be made available to achieve the desired outcomes?

When you are planning to provide a true person centered training program, a successful outcome can be guaranteed by adhering to the following golden rule (Figure 4.2):

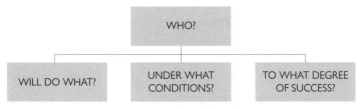

Figure 4.2 The golden rule

Who?

A skilled, knowledgeable clinician is always an educator. When teaching, it is essential to consider who is going to facilitate the training, who is to attend the training (*and this is where I advocate that each and every member of the team, and loved ones, attend any training based around true person centered care*) and who is to support the training, that is, senior management. It is essential that this is clear and precise.

Will do what?

Now you have identified the key people, it is important that you clarify their roles. Essentially, the facilitator is going to deliver the training and the learners will attend. What is equally important is that the role of management support is defined. In what way will that support be demonstrated? Will learners have time to attend? Will they be encouraged to attend and rewarded for doing so? Will any necessary resources be provided? This is a crucial component to a successful outcome of any training. Without this support the whole process is likely to fail.

Under what conditions?

Consideration now has to be given to where the training will be delivered and in what guise. If learners are attending classroom-based sessions, keep them short. Two-and-a-half-hour sessions are long enough. It is essential that learners are supported while theory is delivered at practice level. Think about the learning environment and any equipment you may need. For example, a quiet environment that is light, bright and roomy with a TV and DVD player, flipchart and, if required, PowerPoint are the basic requirements. Ensure you have planned properly and adhere to the timing. Make the learning fun with plenty of opportunity for learners to interact through discussion and short group work exercises.

To what degree of success?

The facilitator, learners and managers must have set, clear outcomes from the training. It is never acceptable to deliver training simply because it will meet a regulatory requirement. It is more important to ensure that no requirement is made in the first place. The ultimate goal of any person centered training has to be to further enhance the quality of life of the people we support. However, this must be combined with enablers who are happy to deliver that level of care. Remembering that this model relies heavily on the family dynamic approach, each person is an important member of the home. To achieve full and complete enrichment a partnership between those living in the home, their loved ones and close friends, and those enabling people to live through their journey is paramount.

To this end, enablers must be equipped with the necessary skills, competence and ability to deliver a truly person centered care program. The four golden rules above will ensure this is achieved.

Psycho-social support strategies

The recommendations put forward in "Always a Last Resort" make clear the need for non-pharmacological interventions when supporting people through the most challenging aspects of their journey. Each and every care home has the responsibility to ensure that this is the case. However, it's not as simple as a doctor saying "I am not going to prescribe medicines until you have exhausted all other avenues." It is necessary that all enablers, including family doctors, are able to suggest what other forms of intervention would be appropriate in each individual case. Following the suggestion, the enabler must have the relevant skills, knowledge, competence and confidence to then apply the intervention. This may be basic counseling techniques that take place each and every day, through to more specialist psychotherapy or cognitive behavior therapy. Whatever strategy is used, training and development are always the key. Is there then an argument for all care homes to have direct access to a qualified and competent psychotherapist who specializes in the field of NCDs? I am of the opinion that this is the case.

In relation to the application of psycho-social support in this field, an appropriate definition is:

> A therapeutic intervention that uses cognitive, cognitive behavior, behavioral and supportive interventions to relieve anxiety and fear, and support people through the many challenges their journey brings.

It has been suggested that people with cognitive change more often than not have impairments in language function and are therefore considered unsuitable for psychotherapy (Duffy 2002). However, this is slightly misleading as the majority of people in the early stages are able to verbally communicate effectively. Even those in the moderate to severe stages of the journey are able to maintain a level of communication, and it is the skill of the clinician that determines the communication tools used for a positive outcome. It is now known that the music center in the brain is separate from the speech and language areas (Broca's and Wernicke's). Therefore, a therapist can communicate effectively by using music as a vehicle.

An evaluation of six 10-week psychotherapy groups for people with cognitive challenges found significant improvement in scores for depression and marginal benefits in anxiety symptoms that were maintained at follow-up (Cheston et al. 2003).

There is evidence that it is possible to apply randomized controlled trial methodology in assessing the impact of a psychotherapeutic approach in people with NCD due to Alzheimer's disease. Although it was found that brief psychotherapy (psychodynamic interpersonal therapy) did not improve scores on any of the key outcome measures, qualitative assessments reported trends toward a subjective benefit for both patients and carers (Burns et al. 2005).

Other work has demonstrated that enhanced psycho-social care can reduce antipsychotic use in care homes without worsening behavioral symptoms (Fossey et al. 2006).

A randomized controlled trial examined the cost effectiveness of a program of cognitive stimulation therapy. The authors found that it was of greater benefit, and might prove to be more cost effective than treatment as usual (Knapp et al. 2006).

In 1997 the American Psychiatric Association produced practice guidelines for the treatment of this patient group. These acknowledged that some clinicians find supportive psychotherapy useful in helping people with mild impairment to adjust to their illness, although there has been little research into its effectiveness.

It is clear that psychotherapy has a major part to play in the delivery of true person centered care, is an area that requires continued study and development, and has the right to attract a level of funding as a valued, active treatment.

In many ways, as a clinician, caregiver, nurse, director or manager, you will regularly use what I term as fundamental psychotherapeutic interventions (FPIs). One example of this is when you sit with an anxious or upset person and offer reassurance and positive engagement; another is where you support an angry person to express their anger through active listening, empathy, genuineness and warmth.

The CAR Approach is useful when providing true person centered care because it encourages everyone, including relatives, professionals and carers, to think about three principal modalities when supporting someone through their journey. These are:

1. communication

2. attitude

3. response.

We will now look at these in more detail and discuss how they fit into the Nightingale Model of Enriched Care.

The CAR Approach

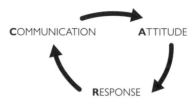

Figure 4.3 The CAR Approach

As you can see from Figure 4.3, the CAR Approach is a cycle of events, and one without the other would be completely ineffectual. The three modalities are interwoven and, when incorporated into the everyday care strategy, are key components to increasing the well-being of each individual.

The term "CAR Approach" itself also helps enablers to maintain a mindset that is positive and encourages individualized care. It takes away that part of our vision that sees only a disability. Instead, it instills a philosophy that allows us all to see the person, and only the person. It is then easier for us to accept that any cognitive change is just a part of who that person really is.

Communication

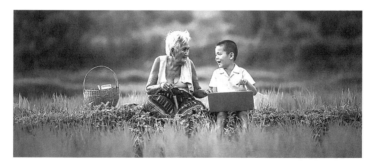

Figure 4.4 Communication

This relates to the way we interact with any one individual. In order to communicate effectively and efficiently, where we achieve a positive outcome to that interaction, we must always consider:

- *Existing skills*, which can be anything from being able to cook their evening meal to being able to point at a chosen meal. It is far more important to establish an existing skill than identify a need. The reason for this is very straightforward: *identifying an existing skill leads to a care plan that can make the identified need less of a need*. By this, I mean the existing skill and ability mean that instead of having to identify that Bill requires assistance to eat his meal, you will be able to identify that Bill is able to put his fork to his mouth if someone sits and eats alongside him. We are therefore increasing Bill's sense of worth and helping him maintain that skill. Very often we see the opposite – Bill will be fed and because of this he is deskilled, further diminished as a person and less likely to have a sense of well-being. By facilitating and supporting this skill, we have effected true person centered care and negated malignant care practice.

- *Competencies* are an essential component for good, positive and successful communication. Competencies are described as skills that are essential to perform certain functions; for example, a clinician needs to be able to use a wide range of skills to communicate with a gentleman who is unable to express himself verbally (expressive dysphasia). Clinician and patient, loved ones, nurses and other persons will always find a method of communication based on the intellectual resources they have at hand. We know for example that music is an excellent vehicle for communicating with people who have lost their competency in verbalization. It will come as no great surprise to many enablers that having a strong relationship with the person, and spending time getting to know them, often lead to successful outcomes in all care areas of delivery. This is because mutual respect develops and each becomes aware of the other's competencies.

- *Knowledge* is power. Every individual comes with a wealth of knowledge and very often a lifetime of experience gained from a varied journey through life. It is essential to remember that having cognitive challenges in no way makes a person less knowledgeable. Here is an example from my clinical work:

I was working with a group of six people, all with varying degrees of dementia. We were doing something called Music and Reminiscence Therapy Incorporating Storytelling, or MaRTiS™, a form of psychotherapy that I devised to make Life Story work more fulfilling for people; more authentic because it truly was *their* life story, as lived and described by each and every individual. We would get together in a room and I would wait until somebody began a conversation. I would then spotlight and zone in on a particular aspect of what the person was saying. This would then lead the group into reminiscing about that particular thing. When the conversation ran dry, we would play some music to trigger more memories. A lady called Mari would attend each and every week. Each and every week she would be assisted from her wheelchair to a comfy armchair, then she would close her eyes and appear to remain locked inside her own world, her own thoughts. I never heard Mari speak until one Wednesday afternoon when the conversation was about Loch Ness and the things that can be found in it. Suddenly, Mari opened her eyes, leaned forward and, in a soft Scottish accent, simply said "salmon." With that, she closed her eyes and leaned back in the chair again. I was amazed that some spark had brought her into my world and, from that moment on, I have stuck to the belief that we should always make one assumption about the people we support: *that the person can always hear and understand everything that is happening around them, everything that is being said about them.*

The type and degree of cognitive change are completely irrelevant when it comes to knowledge. A definition provided by the *Oxford English Dictionary* states that knowledge is an awareness or familiarity gained by experience of a fact or situation. Philosophical debates in general start with Plato's formulation of knowledge as "justified true belief."

Attitude

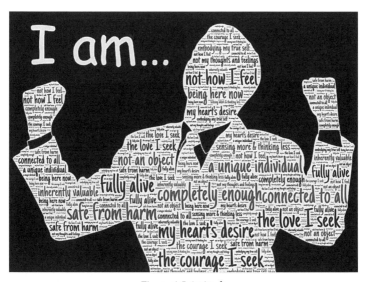

Figure 4.5 Attitude

This relates to the way we interact with the person we are supporting. To ensure our attitude is consistently positive and proactive, we must consider the person's:

- *Holistic function*, which means we look at every aspect of that individual. We support and enable people with their physical, psychological, emotional and spiritual health and well-being. It was during the 1940s that Abraham Maslow first developed his original Hierarchy of Needs (Maslow 1943). Despite its age, it remains an excellent model in relation to dementia care. His original five-stage model is useful here, and easy to apply in the care setting:

1. We start out life with basic *biological and physiological needs*. These are things like sex, food, drink, warmth, sleep and air. Without them we are unable to sustain life, to grow and develop into a fully functioning adult. These things are our central driving system, our motivation to survive. It is essential that we ensure these drives are met as the person works through their journey.

2. Once those basic needs are met, we require *safety*. We need protection, security, order, boundaries, societal norms, laws, etc. Without these, our very existence would be threatened and our ability to thrive in society would be diminished considerably. When somebody moves in to a care home, these needs become even more important and essential. People feel very vulnerable and frightened and we all have a duty to provide an adequate level of care and support that ensures a person's constant need for safety is met. Not to do so will contribute to individual ill-being, malignant care provision and the likelihood of avoidable mortality.

3. When we feel safe and secure, we can then express and receive *love and belongingness*. We have relationships with family members, are able to give and receive affection, work alongside colleagues and have a true sense of who, what and where we are. Developing cognitive challenges

leads to greater dependency on others. This means there is a real danger that people will withdraw into themselves thus impacting in a negative way on relationships. Moving in to a care facility often means a reduction in human contact and physical affection. We must not be afraid to give someone a hug, or hold their hand if they reach out to us. We must do all we can to orientate people and remind them of who, what and where they are.

4. Because we have our fundamental needs and drives met, feel safe and secure and have this overwhelming sense of belonging, our *esteem* allows us to achieve the things we aim for in life. We gain status and responsibility and establish a reputation among our peers and in society as a whole. As cognitive dysfunction takes hold, people are in danger of losing their self-esteem, and very often do. We can reduce this by motivating people, showing them that they really do matter, that they have a true value in society. For example, Tom was a family doctor. He lives in a care home and likes to help in any way he can. Seeking his professional advice and including him gives him increased self-esteem. It appears that when a person loses their role in society, self-esteem becomes low and people begin to feel worthless and useless. By enabling people to maintain some kind of role or function, such as Tom above, or Edith, who for over 50 years worked as a cleaner and likes to help clean the care home in which she now lives, we can help to keep people's esteem at an elevated level, thus reducing the risk of depression and negative feelings about the self.

5. Upon achievement of those things we eventually reach *self-actualization* where we feel we have true personal growth. We have achieved the things we wanted in life and have a true sense of fulfillment. Many people with dementia have self-actualized, while others may not have done so. I will leave you with this thought: *for those who have not, is there any reason why we cannot support them to do so?*

- *Individuality* is so important to each and every one of us. There may be 15 people living in one home. We therefore have 15 different personalities and characters, all with individual strengths, abilities, knowledge, competence and needs. This gives care teams a real challenge in providing true person centered care to each of these people. However, it can be done through a change of attitude and practice – by moving away from task orientated care and embracing the person centered philosophy. Don't rush around like a headless chicken. Take your time. Develop SAPs that allow you to support people through positive engagement. For example, Peter and Jane are married. When Peter went to work this morning he didn't really care whether the bed was made or not. He will fall back into it when he goes to bed tonight. Jane, on the other hand, won't leave for work until the bed is made. If the time comes for either of them to move in to a care home, this desire should be written into their care. Nobody should be rushing around making beds. Respecting individuality is a crucial element in delivering the Dignity in Care Challenge. It reduces the risk of behavior that is a challenge to the service because people continue to feel valued and offered life choices.

- *Lifestyles* are different for many people; they have had different childhoods as well as adulthoods. Many will have shared similar lifestyles too. It is important that group dynamics are built in to the care home strategy. Some people with dementia may find motivation very difficult. For this reason, members of the care and management teams, as well as relatives and friends, can help by completing good, thorough life stories with the person. From this knowledge, you will be able to work out who might get along with whom, thus increasing the potential for the development of good relationships and a sustained, valued lifestyle. We must respect each and every lifestyle, no matter what our own personal feelings may be toward it; we must enable people to continue to live the lifestyle they choose, as difficult and challenging as this may be at times. For example, for whose benefit is it that we expect people to *sleep* at *night* in a *single bed, alone*? Many people don't sleep at night because of their occupation. The majority of people have spent a lifetime sleeping in a double bed, with someone by their side. For whose benefit is it that we expect everyone to sit in a *wing backed chair*? Many people have spent their life chilling out on a sofa. Many things are done for the benefit of the running of the service. What I am asking here is that you challenge that practice; that you think about the real reasons behind uniforms, staff toilets, staff cups, drug trolleys and drug rounds, tea trolleys and tea rounds, laundry trolleys and laundry rounds. Think about how most of your care is delivered by relying on one trolley or the other. It's about removing barriers. It's about removing the *"us and them"* principle and replacing it with *"us."* Consider your own lifestyle and how you would feel if it suddenly changed and you found yourself being cared for. Finally, I will leave you with this thought: *Lifestyles are unique. They are there to be sustained. To disrupt an individual lifestyle is like interfering with nature – disaster will result.*

- *Activities* are something we do from the moment we open our eyes to the moment we close them again. Without activities our very existence would be pointless. Imagine having nothing to do; nobody to interact with; nobody to talk with. You may think that would never happen to the people you support. However, this is not strictly so. In 2007, the Alzheimer's Society in England published a report entitled "Home from Home: A Report Highlighting Opportunities for Improving Standards of Dementia Care in Care Homes," which states that an Alzheimer's Society survey found that the typical person in a home spent only 2 minutes interacting with staff or other residents over a 6-hour period of observation, excluding time spent on care tasks (Alzheimer's Society 2007). The report also stated that research shows that availability of activities and opportunities for occupation is a major determinant of quality of life and affects mortality rates, depression, physical function and behavioral symptoms. I assisted with that document and, from my own experience as a clinical dementia specialist visiting many care services from hospitals to care homes, rather ashamedly have to agree with the statements. It is not a rare incident to see the care and management team busy doing tasks while the very people they are supporting are busy doing nothing. I have no intention of being flippant as I believe this to be due to a lack of adequate training, skills, competence and ability, along with an obvious lack of both human and financial resources. However, having said that, members of the direct care teams do have a part to play in this. We must adopt the attitude that activities are the responsibility of everyone and not simply that of the activities worker. Additionally, if you believe you have a genuine need for more resources in order to meet the everyday needs of people you are supporting, then bring it to the attention of your line manager, but ensure you have sufficient documented evidence beforehand. For example, risk assessments, dependency assessments and behavioral charts. It is then very difficult for funding bodies to argue against your request! It may be useful if you write down all the things you do in a day and compare it to the people that live in the home. What are the differences? How would you feel if you suddenly stopped going to the pub with your mates? Or could no longer spend time with your dog, your horse or anything else that is your main activity away from enabling people in the home?

Response

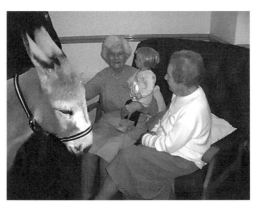

Figure 4.6 Evidence of attachment therapy at its best

By response I mean the way in which we enable people to live positively through their day-to-day challenges by compensating for any losses experienced. The component that makes up the response element of this model is quite simple:

> Providing our response is a positive one, protecting the rights of the individual while respecting their individuality and dignity, there should be no rigid rules to the degree and type of response given.

Consider Figure 4.6. What were your initial thoughts when you first saw it? What key messages does this image send out?

What is happening here is a positive response to a fundamental human need – a need for attachment. Attachment can therefore be defined as:

> A biological function which bases itself on the need for safety, security and protection; attachment promotes survival.

Think about this definition and consider how it is both relevant and applicable to people living in any formal care environment.

Now think about how often a person's need for safety, security and protection are often ignored. What can you do to ensure this is no longer the case with the people you support on a day-to-day basis?

One thing you can do is to speak to each person you walk past. Even if you just say hello and smile at the person. Better still, you could ask how they are and engage in a meaningful conversation, even if it is for a few moments only. What you achieve then is true positive engagement.

When supporting people in a care setting we can always find easy solutions to very complex situations. For example, we can fit child safety gates across bedroom doors to prevent others from entering another's personal space. This is easy and quick – no need for any kind of thought or engagement with the person who wishes to enter the room – but it is inappropriate and a totally unacceptable solution.

What other solutions are there? How would you address this situation in a true person centered way?

It is all about engaging with people; finding out why the person chooses to do that. If people are gainfully employed during their waking hours, this behavior will be avoided.

Focus:

- *On the person, not their diseased brain* – While it is important to have some underpinning knowledge of the pathology of NCDs, it is not crucial to the delivery of true person centered care. Having a cognitive change is only a part of the person. It is far more important to focus on existing skills, knowledge and competence, and celebrate each of those. Contrary to some clinician's views, people can relearn lost skills. Dr Cameron Camp has demonstrated that Montessori techniques can benefit people and I have further adapted this approach to enhance the dining experience of people residing in a care home. Outcomes were very positive and published in the *Journal of Dementia Care* (Nightingale 2011).

Piaget described the Assimilation/Accommodation Theory as:

- *Assimilation* – The process of taking in new information into our previously existing schemas is known as assimilation. The process is somewhat subjective, because we tend to modify experience or information to fit in with our pre-existing beliefs.

- *Accommodation* – Another part of adaptation involves changing or altering our existing schemas in light of new information, a process known as accommodation. Accommodation involves altering existing schemas, or ideas, as a result of new information or new experiences. New schemas may also be developed during this process. Therefore, if one can ride a push bike, those basic skills can be adapted to ride a motorbike.

In my work, I looked at a more positive dining experience. Participants spent 30 minutes on Montessori-based activities before having 15 minutes to make their way to the dining area. The idea was based on repetitive actions. During the activities, the participants transferred cotton wool balls from a container to a bun tray with colored dots. They used their tongues to do this. On having their meal, they eventually continued to use those skills while eating their meal. Previous to this, they had been fully supported during their meals by support staff who had been feeding each person. This small but effective pilot study demonstrates that people with dementia can possibly relearn skills that have been lost (Nightingale 2011).

The question is:

Have those skills been lost due to the effects of the cognitive deficit itself, and the repetitive activity has laid down new neuronal pathways? Or, was the skill lost because enablers found it more convenient and less time-consuming to simply feed people?

I will leave it to each individual reader to think about that question and search for the appropriate answer!

- *On their emotions and understandings, not memory losses* – There can be no argument that as long as a person exists, he or she will always be able to experience emotions. This is why doll therapy, pet therapy and true human contact result in positive well-being for each person. As I identified above, always assume that the person is able to understand everything that is being said around them and everything that is being done with them. To focus on a person's losses is detrimental to their health and well-being. The process known as Dementia Care

Mapping would identify this as malignant, so avoid it. (Dementia Care Mapping is an established approach to achieving and embedding person centered care for people living with dementia. It was developed at the Bradford Centre for Applied Dementia Studies and is the brainchild of the late Professor Tom Kitwood.) If the person is anxious and distressed about memory loss, then you must support him or her through that experience. If anger or frustration is expressed, this must be permitted. Very often we see enablers use distraction techniques to try and resolve an expression of anger or frustration. Ask yourself this question: "If my wallet were stolen, would I want someone to talk to me about the weather and offer me a cup of tea?" Remember that people living in a care home have lost their wallets, and much, much more besides. Thus, people have a right to be angry but also have a right to be supported to express that anger in a way that is not destructive or harmful to that person or to others. What do you do to express your anger and frustration? How did the person in question express theirs before cognitive change and prior to living in the care home? It is crucial to find out. Only then are you in a position to support that person as they express their emotions and current understanding of present events.

- *On the person within the context of a marriage or family* – Part of this model considers family dynamics as crucial to true person centered care. We have looked at this earlier in the book (see p.60–61); therefore, I shall simply remind you to ensure we are always working toward a PFD experience with each and every person we support on a day-to-day basis.

- *On the person within a wider society and its values* – In order to have a successful outcome from the provision of residential or nursing home care, the service and all its activities must be fully inclusive of society as a whole. Managers and members of the direct care teams must look outside of the care services to forge links with others. One example is to utilize spare rooms and resources for things like a local artist to hold a gallery there for a couple of days. Another is to support local business and networking groups in holding their monthly breakfast meetings there. By doing these things you are able to raise the profile of the home and fully include it in other things that happen in the community. I can hear people saying "We can't do that. Someone in authority somewhere will have something to say," etc. Not necessarily so – something I remember from a presentation I once attended is that a problem is only ever a solution in disguise! So, put your thinking caps on and truly embrace your local community and get involved with all that is happening in it.

This model is practical; it works in clinical practice. It will work in practice when we all embrace and apply it in our roles. The individual themselves, their loved ones and friends, doctors, nurses, social workers, directors, care workers, managers, social workers, commissioning bodies and regulators all have a part to play.

Chapter 5

Using the Nightingale Dementia Triangle in Clinical Practice

This model is based on my clinical belief that the symptoms of any NCD are exacerbated by two emotional fuels: fear and anxiety. When I visit a patient in their family home, care home or hospital, or when they come to my office, these emotions are difficult to miss. By observing an individual's behavior and language, it is often easy to establish the nature of their particular negative emotional state. People who are in the early stages of their journey often cannot identify why they feel the way they do, but they can feel the changes within their mind and body. This fundamental model assists the clinician in helping the patient understand how those emotions can be changed.

Psychology defines fear as "the unpleasant emotional state consisting of psychological and psychophysiological responses to a real external threat or danger" and anxiety as "an emotion characterized by feelings of tension, worried thoughts and physical changes like increased blood pressure."

If we consider those two definitions in relation to people living with an NCD it is easy to see how their personhood can be stripped away with ease. Imagine having a short-term memory dysfunction such that each morning when you wake, you have no idea where you are. It's the same

environment you have lived in for the past 40 years, but
you don't recognize it. Fear and anxiety are immediately
intensified. The person you wake up next to is a total stranger,
though you have woken up next to that person for the past
40 years. The fear and anxiety have now been exacerbated
even further. Your immediate response is to get up and run
away, but you cannot because you don't know where you
would run to. The person next to you wakes up and reaches
out to kiss you. They speak but you have no idea what
they are saying. They get up and leave the bedroom. A few
moments later, someone in a uniform enters and indicates
for you to get dressed. They make the bed and leave. Now
your fear and anxiety has taken control of your entire being.
This is a feeling you are going to experience throughout the
day – a perpetual darkness that is everlasting. Everything
around you is forever changing, something I refer to as "each
minute different, everything always new." The real enemies
are not Alzheimer's disease or other cognitive change agents,
but fear and anxiety. Once this is addressed and managed as
effectively as possible, the person can begin to grow again
and their confidence and self-esteem will re-emerge like the
phoenix rising from the ashes. They are no longer oppressed
by these uninvited guests.

In Chapter 3 we looked at how hypnosis as a therapy
can be beneficial. In this chapter I will use a real live case
study, with names and details changed to protect anonymity
and patient–doctor confidentiality, to demonstrate how the
application of this model can further improve outcomes
from any modality of therapy.

CASE STUDY

Carole is 82 years old with a diagnosis of vascular NCD. She has
resided in a small care home for almost 4 months. She has no
known family and had been living alone until she was no longer

able to do so due to cognitive decline. Considering her advanced years, she is physically healthy and has no problems with her mobility, hearing or sight. However, Carole's cognitive change has led to an inability to speak apart from a low moaning sound that she produces at times of stress. Other than this Broca's (expressive) dysphasia, caused by a cerebrovascular accident she had 12 months previous to moving to her new home, she lives in her own silent world where she has withdrawn from her external environment. Despite this, Carole has no difficulty understanding what others are saying to her, so there is no evidence of receptive dysphasia.

The past few nights, Carole has been waking up and presenting with behaviors that are new for her. She opens her wardrobe and removes all her clothes. She pulls out drawers in her room and rummages through them. She then starts to produce the low moaning sound that gets louder and louder as she bangs on doors. The staff noted that her facial expressions and body language changed dramatically during these events. Her GP had ruled out anything physical and had referred her to me.

The care home has very little background information about Carole and her Life Story book consisted of only one page. Yes, one page of life for someone who has lived for eight decades. I knew it was going to be complicated to identify the underlying causes of this behavior, but identify it I would.

The only way I was going to be able to observe this behavior directly was through physical presence at the care home when Carole was in bed. She usually retired at about 10pm so I ensured I was there 2 hours earlier with an ABC Recording Chart (Antecedent, Behavior and Consequence). An *antecedent* is something that comes before a particular behavior. A *behavior* is anything an individual does and a *consequence* is something that follows that behavior. It is imperative that this three-part observation record be completed accurately at the exact time a particular behavior is expressed.

Table 5.1 Carole's completed ABC Recording Chart

Date	Time	Environment	Antecedent	Behavior	Consequence	Signature
2/4/2018	8.45pm	Lounge	All six people living in the house had just finished watching a film on TV	Carole started to look around the room. She began to tap her fingers on the arm of the chair	Care assistant Sally asked Carole if she wanted some tea and toast. Took her by the hand and led her to the dining room	DJN
2/4/2018	9.15pm	Dining room	Carole was finishing her supper	She began to feel and look under the table	Care assistant Sally asked Carole if she would like to get ready for bed and took her by the hand. They left and headed to the bathroom	DJN
2/4/2018	10.50pm	Carole's bedroom	Carole was in bed	She could be heard moaning quietly from where I was sitting in the hallway	No action was taken as I wanted to observe any further behavior	DJN
2/4/2018	10.55pm	Carole's bedroom	Carole was walking around her room	She could be heard banging cupboard and wardrobe doors	Sally and I entered her bedroom and saw she was clearly distressed. She was anxious and looked afraid. Sally sat with her and offered reassurance	DJN

On assessing Carole's behavior it became apparent that she was seeking something. Given her age and my experience of this sort of behavior pattern, I suspected she was possibly looking for a lost child. The very next morning I spoke with her GP who did some digging up of historical medical notes and discovered that Carole had lost an 18-month-old daughter due to polio when she was 23.

With that information in hand, the solution was relatively straightforward: doll therapy. In a paper published in *Frontiers in Psychology*, Rita Pezzati et al. (2014, p.342) stated that doll therapy "is a non-pharmacological intervention aimed at reducing behavioral and psychological disorders in institutionalized patients with dementia." My preference would always be inclusion of reality, and in this case it would be interaction between children and Carole. However, this could be organized at a later date, as an immediate intervention was necessary to address her current psychological trauma.

Later that day, I met with Carole and the care home team, including the owner/manager, to develop a SAP that would address the issue without further delay. First, we considered the Nightingale Dementia Triangle and how it was relevant to Carole.

Carole appears to be in a positive state of well-being during most parts of the day (it is important that we have the mindset that she "appears" to be in a positive state as we can never know what her exact thoughts are as the day progresses). What we do know as fact is that at night time she searches for something lost. This is a time when dementia is in control of her very being; it is a time when dementia is feeding on an abundance of fear and anxiety. As such, Carole is diminished as an individual and her personhood compromised.

In Figure 5.1, we see *dementia* as the central player: the commander over Carole's life and everything that happens. Dementia has two allies: *fear* and *anxiety*. Together, they form the Dementia Triangle that fuels the disease and reduces every aspect of her quality of life. This person, Carole, is slowly diminishing; becoming a shrinking violet with reduced confidence and self-esteem; withdrawing into a shell; becoming a shadow of her former self. Night after night, as a person, Carole lives in constant fear. Every action is surrounded by high states of anxiety. Unless, through therapy, things change, Carole, the person, will not be able to live well with dementia. Gradually, she will become more and more diminished, more and more disempowered until end of life comes, and this will come much quicker than it needs to.

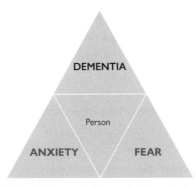

Figure 5.1 The Nightingale Dementia Triangle showing the negative impact of dementia on Carole prior to doll therapy

SAP

Though the issue for Carole was causing her severe trauma due to increased levels of fear and anxiety, we all agreed that the solution was not complex. First, we introduced a life-like baby (one that is used specifically in doll therapy) to Carole.

Initially Carole turned away, so we left the baby on the chair and continued discussing the plan. After only a few moments, Carole picked up the baby and cradled her in her arms. She smiled!

We then asked Carole if she would like us to put a cot in her bedroom for the baby. There was no hesitation. She stood and led the way.

The cot was placed next to Carole's bed and she instantly placed the baby in the cot and covered her with a blanket. She looked contented and her facial expression, which was normally absent of smiles and softness, changed in a positive way. She looked serene, at peace.

The SAP put Carole at the heart of this doll therapy intervention. She was in charge of caring for the baby and nobody interfered with her responsibility. Already, her identity as a "mum" was back, and thus her personhood had meaning again.

That night, when Carole went to bed, we realized we had extinguished the behavior of waking and searching: a behavior that not only awoke the symptoms of her cognitive change, but also the fear and anxiety. It was now gone. Carole slept through the night and, when the care assistant peeked in to check on her at midnight, she was fast asleep, the baby in her arms.

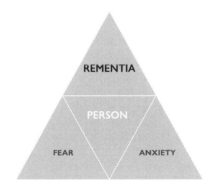

Figure 5.2 The Nightingale Dementia Triangle showing the positive impact of therapy for Carole

Now we have supported Carole through an appropriate intervention, in this case, doll therapy, the triangle has changed. It is at this juncture that the *person* and the care team have waged war against *fear* and *anxiety*. *Dementia* is no longer the commander. Instead, the person has taken center stage. We have managed to transform a malignant life of dementia into a productive life of *rementia*. Rementia is defined as "the regaining of lost cognitive functional abilities." Now the person once again has confidence and self-esteem, empowerment and is more able to take control over her own life. Personhood has returned.

The Dementia Triangle can be used in both straightforward cases such as the one described and more complex cases. The object is always the same: to turn dementia into rementia; to empower the person and cut off the nutrition that feeds fear and anxiety. At the time of writing, Carole continues to live well with her challenges and both loves and cares for the baby like any mother would.

Chapter 6

The Clinical and Clinician's Environment

There is much focus on the living environment and how it impacts on the quality of life of people living with NCDs. For example, the Dementia Development Centre at the University of Stirling has been the leader on designing services for over 25 years.

Imagine that over your lifetime your brain has developed something called an ecological inventory. This is made up of environmental cues and images. An example of this is when one asks for directions you may be instructed to "turn left at the White Horse pub and then second right after the church. You will see a post box on the corner. That's where you need to turn." Your environmental cues are made up of things like landmarks, street signs, post boxes, telephone kiosks and bus stops. It is therefore crucial that people living with an NCD continue to be exposed to such cues to aid orientation. There are ecological inventory tools that can be used to teach functional skills that are necessary in natural environments.

Joost van Hoof et al. (2010) discuss "Environmental interventions and the design of homes for older adults with dementia" in an article published in the *American Journal of Alzheimer's Disease and Other Dementias*. In my early days as the dementia specialist for Highfield Care in 2002 I began to implement environmental change in the nursing homes. Thus, this area of dementia care is not a new one.

However, what of our own environment as clinicians? What can we do that will alter our own external environment in order to have the best positive impact on patients visiting our office or clinic? This chapter aims to answer that question, along with suggesting strategies to change our own psychological belief systems that influence clinical conceptions to ensure a positive, engaging and meaningful consultation. By addressing our professional and personal self, we can ensure that the delivery of a diagnosis (es) and treatment/therapy is done in a structured and positive way.

Clinical/Office Environment

The very moment somebody living with an NCD leaves their familiar environment, there is a huge risk that their fear and anxiety levels, the nutrition that fuels their BPSD, will begin to intensify. Combined with the knowledge the person is visiting a dentist, GP, consultant or therapist, it is probable the patient is heading toward unsafe levels of those fuels. One of the challenges faced by most people with a primary NCD is disorientation to time and place. If I were to ask someone who is not experiencing cognitive decline to tell me the time without looking at a watch or clock they would come very close. However, if I were to ask one of my patients that very same question it may be difficult for them to come anywhere close.

Here are a few things you can do to have an immediate positive impact on the patient's fear, anxiety and stress levels when they arrive:

- Music has the inherent ability to decrease the psychobiological response to stress and anxiety. Therefore, ensure you have the music "Weightless" by Marconi Union playing in the reception area. Neuroscience has proven that this particular music reduces overall anxiety by 65 percent with a 35 percent reduction in patients' usual physiological resting states as shown in research conducted by Dr David Lewis-Hodgson of Mindlab International based in Brighton. To help even further, request that the patient be exposed to "Weightless" during their journey to the office or clinic. By doing this, you are already one step ahead, and this makes a huge difference to the outcomes of the consultation or therapy. We have learned that the music center of the brain is not part of the Broca's or Wernicke's areas. A study carried out by the Massachusetts Institute of Technology mathematically analyzed scans of the auditory cortex and grouped clusters of brain cells with similar activation patterns, thus identifying neural pathways that react exclusively to the sound of music (Norman-Haignere 2015). This explains why music is one of the most successful communication vehicles for people when they have severe damage to the speech and language centers of the brain.

- Use the color blue in your waiting room and consulting/therapy office. It is tranquil and calming and has an amazing ability to help manage stress. A very soothing color, blue helps to reduce the heart rate, lower blood pressure and reduce anxiety. A soft, neutral shade of blue will yield the best results. Avoid the color red as much as possible. Not just in decoration but also in relation to uniforms (and instruments if you are a dentist). Red has been shown to increase anxiety and is often interpreted by the brain as "danger," something to avoid or stay away from. It enhances the metabolism, increases respiration rate and raises blood pressure.

- Unless you are a sole practitioner, ensure you allocate one of the team to support the patient from the moment they arrive. Have a number of interactive activities available that will provide meaningful and engaging occupation until you are ready to meet with the individual. This will help to keep the person distracted and calm. Every interaction is aimed at keeping negative emotions at bay while encouraging a positive mindset.

Those are three fundamental ways in which you can reduce the fear and anxiety of someone living with an NCD who has a need to visit your office or clinic. As a personal preference I would much rather do a home visit. However, this isn't always possible or practical, so implementing these suggestions is the second best option.

Staff Training and Development

It is crucial that all the staff working in your office or clinic have at least a basic understanding of the most common types of NCDs and how they impact on the individual. What is especially important is knowing how to engage positively with the patient and their caregiver. Remember, it doesn't matter who comes into contact with them, they are now part of that unique journey and, in this case, your staff team are a key component in keeping fear and anxiety levels at a bare minimum.

Unless you work solely on your own, doctors' offices, hospitals, clinics and therapist offices can be very busy with an abundance of activity going on. This can be distressing for an individual with an NCD and a skilled team can ensure the individual remains unaffected by all the "buzz" around them.

It is important that every person feels included in normality, or, the phrase I have coined to describe this, "inclusion of reality" while they are assisted to maintain their levels of fear, anxiety and stress within safe parameters. Among other things, training must include communication strategies, the environment and positive engagement.

Specific to Dental Offices

In addition to the things mentioned earlier in this chapter, there are a few additional strategies specific to dentists and dental staff that will ensure a more patient centered visit and outcome to treatment. These are:

- Ensure the dental assistant communicates with the patient throughout the entire dental process. Choose a subject that interests the patient and communicate at a level the person understands. You can even sing if you like – remember what we said about the power and effects of music?

- The dentist or oral hygienist carrying out the dental work should always explain what is happening – adhere to the motto that "the patient can hear and understand everything that is being said to them and everything that is being done." By doing that, you are respecting and valuing the individual to a degree that supports every other strategy aimed at reassurance.

- The music being played in the reception area should also be filtered through to the dental room so it can be heard in the background.

- Dental staff need to be aware of a behavior known in psychology as mirroring. This is the subconscious replication of another person's non-verbal signals. Be attuned to your own body language so you only convey positive messages and have an awareness of your emotional, or cognitive, empathy.

- If need be, let the person see the instruments you are going to use prior to using them. Explain what it is and how it works.

- Schedule more time for any procedures you are going to carry out on your patient.

All therapy and procedures are very often stressful for most people; hence the term "white coat hypertension," which is a syndrome whereby a patient's feeling of anxiety in a clinical environment results in abnormally high blood pressure. It is therefore in everyone's best interests to take as much proactive action as possible in order to reduce these risks, which are far greater in those living with an NCD.

Changing Our Clinical Psychological Belief Systems

Who was it who said the doctor knows best? Yes, it was the doctor! In 2009, Alan Johnson, the then Health Secretary at Westminster, launched an NHS Constitution that was aimed at bringing an end to a lifetime where "doctor knows best."

This fits well with all the strategies that have since been developed to support people who are living with an NCD. Doctors must tell patients which medical treatments and options are available and let them decide for themselves.

It is now time to challenge ourselves and our own conceptions about the care, support and advice we offer to those whose journey we play a part in.

The *Oxford English Dictionary* defines psychological as "Of, affecting, or arising in the mind; related to the mental and emotional state of a person" and a belief system as "a set of principles or tenets which together form the basis of a religion, philosophy or moral code." If we marry these definitions together we can propose that the psychological belief system of a clinician is a *mental and emotional belief in a philosophy grounded on one's own principles and biases*.

If this is the case, then they are unique to each individual clinician, no matter what field one specializes in. As a clinical dementia specialist I need to be open to many ideas and must be flexible in both my expectancy and personal bias. If this is so for me, then this is also the case for others.

Let us consider a conversation I recently had with a colleague about NCDs in childhood. She was of the opinion that disorders such as Nieman–Pick's type C and Batten disease are so rare that they don't warrant too much attention, and that the parents of such children require no additional support outside of palliative or end-of-life care. This was her mental and emotional belief grounded in her own principles and biases. From a clinical viewpoint it is neither right nor wrong, but if you are the parents of such a child then it would be distressing to hear her express such a belief. The best way of altering this perception is through reflective practice, recorded role play and feedback.

Reflective practice is a way of studying your own experiences to improve the way you work. It is very useful for health professionals who want to carry on learning throughout their lives. The act of reflection is a great way to increase confidence and become a more proactive and qualified professional. Additionally, it provides the clinician with an opportunity to review the impact their practice has on those receiving their professional service, be it medical, nursing, psychology, psychotherapy, psychiatry or other form of therapy.

Role play is about acting out or performing the part of a person or character; for example, as a technique in training as a psychotherapist, hypnotherapist, psychiatrist, registered nurse or other professional.

Feedback, in this case, refers to the information about reactions to a scenario played out by clinicians in order to identify areas for improvement and development.

CASE STUDY

Carla has been a clinical psychologist and hypnotherapist for over 20 years. Recently she attended a training program aimed at using hypno-psychotherapy with people who have a primary NCD.

As primary NCDs are degenerative Carla has always believed nothing can be done to change that; her professional view has always been that only medication will help address the BPSD. For this reason, she has never been proactive in her practice.

During this course, Carla was exposed to Kolb's experiential learning theory (Kolb and Kolb 2012), which functions on two levels. These are a four-stage cycle of learning (Figure 6.1) and four separate learning styles (Figure 6.2).

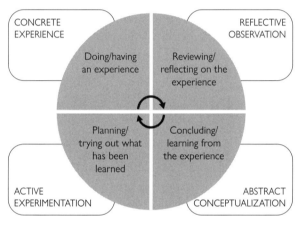

Figure 6.1 The four-stage cycle of learning

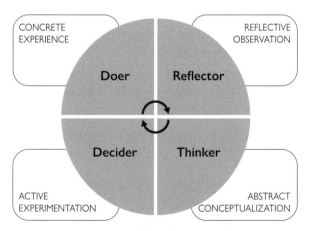

Figure 6.2 The four learning styles

Carla's own learning style was that of a doer following a concrete experience. The aim of reflective practice for her was to take her learning style, provide a concrete experience through role play and feedback what she had learned.

The role play scenario focused on use of the Nightingale Dementia Triangle we discussed in Chapter 5 as an alternative to prescribing antipsychotic medicine to manage severe anxiety disorder. It was the first time Carla had come across this therapy concept. A fellow learner played the role of Gareth, a 73-year-old retired police officer who was living with a mixed NCD (in this case, both NCD due to Alzheimer's disease and NCD with Lewy bodies). He experiences both severe anxiety and regular visual hallucinations, and the use of antipsychotic medicine in such cases can lead to premature mortality. The aim of this role play exercise was to change the dementia to rementia and manage the anxiety without resorting to use of medication. Carla provided a session of hypno-psychotherapy with Gareth and discovered he was still affected by an incident that happened toward the end of his career as a police inspector. She was now faced with treating the symptoms of post-traumatic stress disorder, realizing that it was this that was the issue and nothing to do with Alzheimer's disease or Lewy body.

Reflecting on the role play experience Carla agreed that as clinicians we must always uncover the cause of symptoms as opposed to attributing them to the NCD a person is living with. Her feedback demonstrated a shift in her own belief system and clinical conceptions.

It is crucial that we retain an open mind when assessing and treating people in order that they receive the best we can offer to ensure their journey is supported in a positive manner. As clinicians we must reach inside our professional self and allow change in perception and conception even during a consultation or when delivering therapy. Whether you are a clinical dementia specialist, GP, hypnotherapist, psychotherapist, admiral nurse or other clinician, the formula of reflective practice + role play + feedback can help you modify your belief systems and biases to ensure that your patient receives true person centered care.

Chapter 7

Neuro Linguistic Programming with People Living with a Neurocognitive Disorder

Neuro linguistic programming (NLP) is an approach to communication, personal development and psychotherapy that was created in the 1970s at the University of California, Santa Cruz, by Richard Bandler and John Grinder. The technique relates thoughts, language and patterns of behavior learned through experience to specific outcomes. NLP is a fail free therapy, which makes it ideal for people who are living with an NCD. *Neuro* relates to the interaction between body and mind, while *linguistic* is the clues that can be gained as to the way an individual thinks based on their chosen use of language. Finally, *programming* is the study of the patterns of speaking and the behavior that are adopted in everyday life.

Grinder is a linguist and Bandler an information scientist and mathematician, and their first book on the subject, *Structure of Magic: A Book about Language of Therapy*, was published in 1975 (Bandler and Grinder 1975). Much of the content of this book focuses on the work of Fritz Perls, a noted German psychiatrist and psychotherapist, who developed an approach called Gestalt therapy; Milton Erikson, an American psychiatrist and psychologist, who specialized in medical hypnosis and family therapy;

and Virginia Satir, an American therapist and author, who was known for her approach to family therapy and family reconstruction therapy.

NLP is widely used in counseling, medicine, law, business, the performing arts, sport, the military and education and, because of the way it works, it has much value as a therapy for people on their journey through cognitive change. For example, NLP suggests there are six logical levels of change, and you will see that each one of them has some relevance to the unique journey being lived by everyone with an NCD.

1. *Purpose and spirituality*, which can be the involvement in something much larger than oneself such as global warming. NLP describes this as the highest level of change. I will relate this level of change to a patient with frontotemporal lobar degeneration with progressive non-fluent aphasia. This person developed an amazing talent to paint only after onset of his journey. This gave him so much more purpose.

2. *Identity*, which is described as how a person perceives themselves to be and is inclusive of the responsibilities and roles they have played throughout their life. As we know, there is a risk of their personhood being stolen during their journey unless steps are taken to maintain a level of responsibility and roles.

3. *Beliefs and values* relates to a person's personal belief system and the things that matter most. Carl Jung once described the personality as a "unique, dynamic, ever changing self," which is a great phrase that reminds us of how our belief systems and values continue to grow and change throughout our lifetime. Those living with an NCD may have their personality affected early in their journey, and it may be this that has an influence on their changing values.

4. *Capabilities and skills* relate to what a person can do. As we have learned from previous chapters in this book, one of the most important aspects of supporting people living with an NCD is to focus on their existing capabilities and skills.

5. *Behaviors* are the specific actions people perform, with each action being a form of communication. Very often, when we are providing any form of therapy to people who are on their final stage of their journey, the art of interpreting body language at a conscious level becomes crucial as a successful form of communication.

6. *Environment* is described in NLP as the lowest level of change. It relates to one's setting, including other people. In Chapter 6 we saw how the environment impacts on the person's journey, and its importance in influencing levels of fear and anxiety.

The reader will see the relevance of how these principles relate to those who are living with an NCD, and Figure 7.1 indicates their connection to true person centered care. The levels of change can be at any time and in any order, but the significance is that each and every change has an impact. As clinicians and therapists, it is our responsibility to ensure all impacts due to change are positive.

In short, NLP is a therapy that encourages a change in thoughts and behaviors aimed at achieving positive outcomes for the person. It is founded on the idea that people operate via internal maps of the world that they learn through sensory experience and relies on the reprogramming of the nervous system through the use of language.

For people living with an NCD, this therapy can be beneficial in the following ways:

- It helps the person manage their own internal state – we know how fear and anxiety impact on the individual. Other internal states such as stress, panic, lowered confidence and self-esteem, withdrawal into self and the inability to hold a state of internal calm also lead to a state of ill-being. The use of some NLP techniques can change this so the person begins to enjoy a state of well-being.

- It helps the person remain resourceful during stressful times – no matter how far along the individual is in their journey, various resources, tools, coping strategies and skills built from past experience still remain. Techniques of NLP can help the person use these resources to improve their day-to-day quality of life.

- It gives the person behavioral flexibility in stressful situations – imagine a patient who has recently moved into a care home or memory care community, where the doors may be locked and he or she has no way of getting out. A feeling of imprisonment or a belief that one has been entrapped increases fear and anxiety and may lead to rage. Banging on doors and windows as a message to "let me out of here" is a likely outcome. Of course, this should never happen in the first place; however, in reality, we know it does. To this day I continue to hear people refer to the "lock down unit," which, in itself, is a personal detractor. NLP can help a person change their behavioral responses, again by using the skills and abilities they are using to exhibit the behavior of banging on doors and windows.

- It increases the ability to learn new material – we know, through neuroplasticity and some Montessori-type activities, people can relearn lost skills. NLP can help people relearn through their own learning style. A person may learn best through their visual senses, for example, so mirroring would be the ideal way to help them relearn. An example of this would be sitting down with someone who sees the food on their plate but has forgotten how to get it from there into their mouth. Mirror neurons work by literally "mirroring" the behavior of others through expectation that a particular action will occur. This is based on experience. If I sit opposite you and wave a bottle of water around randomly, your mirror neurons will remain inactive. However, if I bring the water bottle to my lips, your experience tells you I am going to drink from it and your mirror neurons will wake and fire. Thus, in the case of "mirror" eating, the demonstrator will eat and encourage the other person to copy, or mimic, that behavior. As the brain has learned the likely action that is about to take place, the mirror neuron fires. Somebody else may learn better through their auditory senses where only a verbal reminder is necessary. An example of this would be asking Alice, who may have forgotten a sequence, to put on her blouse, then her cardigan. Another way may be through the kinesthetic sense, where a person relearns something from a hands-on experience such as the Montessori principles.

As we can see, the use of NLP supports all that we do in terms of delivering true person centered care and person focused therapy. Through the use of a case study I will demonstrate how we can help a lady who experiences severe panic attacks on a regular basis.

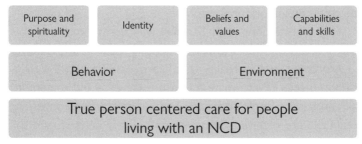

Figure 7.1 The six levels of change described in NLP and the relevance to people living with an NCD

CASE STUDY

Caroline is 72 years of age with a diagnosis of NCD due to Alzheimer's disease. She is married, living at home with her husband John, and they are both retired from running their own engineering company. They have no children. Caroline has lived with panic attacks for as long as she can remember, however, over the past 6 months they have grown more severe and more regular.

The Mayo Clinic states that panic attacks are sudden episodes of intense fear that triggers severe physical reactions when there is no real danger or apparent cause. They can be very frightening and, when they do occur, people believe they are losing control, having a heart attack or even dying.

Caroline's attacks come on suddenly, without warning, at no given time and in any environment or situation. People may differ in their experience and symptomology can also be varied. Caroline's typical symptoms are an increased rapid heart rate, shaking, hot flashes, headache and feelings of detachment.

Though I was not able to uncover the trigger for these panic attacks, I believe there may have been some genetic disposition as both her sister and mother experienced them throughout their lifetime. What was apparent, and the reason for her referral to me by her GP, was that since the onset of her cognitive change the attacks had grown more intense and were now happening once every few days. With the National Institute for Health and Care Excellence (NICE) Guidelines recommending that some form of counseling be preferred over medication (Clark 2011), her GP was reluctant to prescribe a benzodiazepine or antidepressant.

My first meeting with Caroline was spent explaining how the brain actually takes in what it is being fed from the external environment, or the reality that it processes. From the many million pieces of information that it receives – and remember, all the senses come into play here – only a fraction of the real facts are received. Some are completely deleted (and this is further exacerbated by damage to, and the shrinking of,

Caroline's hippocampus); others are distorted while the brain generalizes other information. It is as though the brain reads a paragraph of a story but only accepts half the facts and makes up the rest. So, the symptoms of Caroline's panic attacks are not harmful. The damage comes from her own interpretation of those symptoms, such as "I'm going to have a heart attack" or "I'm going to die from this." This is the story that she tells herself based on her own belief.

Additionally, I needed to learn about her personality and learning style. It turned out she had a great sense of humor, was very intelligent and optimistic. She was a risk taker and a sponge when it came to learning anything new. Despite her assertive nature she had always allowed her panic disorder to get the better of her. She was a visual person when it came to learning new skills or material.

On average, the human concentration span is approximately 8 seconds, which has fallen from 12 seconds since the year 2000. Compare this to the concentration span of a goldfish, which is 9 seconds! Out of all the information available to Caroline's brain, and there is now more information available to the human race than there has ever been before, she will always find something to support her beliefs. So, the things we are tuned in to, and this could be anything, but for Caroline it is the panic attacks and the symptoms that accompany them, are the things the brain focuses on. Her world was shrinking day by day. Her personhood was collapsing and her quality of life was extremely poor. She was finding herself in a state of ill-being for much longer periods of time.

My next meeting with Caroline was to utilize NLP, with the aim of altering her story, thus changing her belief around these panic attacks and their meaning. Her experiences of panic attacks had created her thought pattern identification, which had led her to develop the choices she opted for in responding to the attacks. Caroline's pattern recognition in relation to her response to this panic disorder remains stored in her brain, which means it can be accessed and changed. What was happening was her response to her map of reality and not reality itself. By getting her to recognize and accept that all meaning is subjective – that it is the way she interprets her symptoms to indicate she is having a panic attack – meant she was able to change it. As always in therapy I shared the Dementia Triangle with Caroline and we developed a SAP.

There is the past, the present and the future. For some people, the future is directly in front of them; for others it may be to the left or right. Caroline indicated her future was directly in front of her (at this critical point it is always important to remember that for most people living with an NCD, the present is what matters more than anything, and we can use this to our advantage when treating panic attacks through NLP). On testing, I reaffirmed that she was a very visual person and that GVI was something she didn't have a problem with. I drew a timeline on a huge sheet of paper with focus on the *present* and asked her to imagine hovering over that timeline and observing her inner self having a severe panic attack (this is the event). She was safe because she was hovering above her inner self, therefore she was in control of *it* and *it* could never be in control of her. She was able to see that the symptoms of increased rapid heart rate, shaking, hot flashes, headache and feelings of detachment could mean something totally different, something pleasurable and enjoyable. I then asked her to go beyond the event, after it was over, turn and look at its outcomes. I asked her to tell me something pleasurable she had experienced in the past that gave her the feelings of increased rapid heart rate, shaking and hot flashes – her answer was a ride at the funfair. We repeated this a number of times until her anxiety based around panic attacks decreased so much I was able to introduce the swish technique.

The way I used this procedure with Caroline was to ask her to close her eyes and imagine a huge TV screen.

> Now, watch yourself having a panic attack – be in the moment. Really see yourself experiencing that event and quickly change your viewing to another larger TV screen where you create an

image of what it's like to *never* have a panic attack again. Clear of anxiety. Clear of fear. Smile to yourself. Give a little giggle at something you find really funny. Be in that moment. The other TV screen has shrunk so much you can't see the image. All you see is yourself, panic attack free. Anxiety free.

The most important component of this technique is the speed with which it evolves. Though it very often has a positive impact after only one session, with people experiencing cognitive change it may take two or three sessions.

For Caroline, our session was recorded so she could watch it whenever she needed to do so. Her panic attacks reduced significantly (though they did not cease completely) and, as a result, her quality of life and well-being improved immensely. There was no need for anti-anxiety medicine and she carried a card around with her for the times she did have a panic attack. It read "Everything is okay. I'm in control. This is just a passing moment. I'm safe. I'm in control of my breathing."

Caroline's husband learned the swish technique and used it with her a few times a week as both an aide memoire and an exercise for continued change to her thought patterns.

As we learn more about the negative impact living with an NCD has on an individual, we also learn more about the positive impact various therapies can have, with NLP being just one such therapy.

Chapter 8

The Use of Cognitive Behavior Therapy with People Living with a Neurocognitive Disorder

Cognitive behavior therapy (CBT) is a short-term goal orientated form of psychotherapy. With this technique, the client is encouraged and expected to take a hands-on approach to addressing their psychological problems in order to seek a solution. The ultimate goal is to change negative thoughts and images into more positive ones, thus altering the outcomes from such thinking.

The CBT approach was pioneered by Dr Aaron Beck, a psychiatrist, in the 1960s. At the time of writing, now 97, Dr Beck remains the Professor Emeritus in the Department of Psychiatry at the University of Pennsylvania. He is also the President Emeritus of the Beck Institute for CBT, which he set up in 1994 with his psychologist daughter Dr Judith Beck.

I have used CBT extensively in my practice both as a general psychotherapist and clinical dementia specialist. The beauty of CBT is that it can be used in conjunction with other therapies such as hypno-psychotherapy and NLP.

The way a cognitive behavior therapist works is to assess the person's thoughts, moods, behaviors, biology and environment to help understand the origin of the problem(s). These five areas are interconnected, with each part influencing the others. It places particular emphasis on identifying and evaluating thoughts and on behavioral change. As a clinician and practitioner of CBT, I do not necessarily believe that thoughts cause all problems. However, thoughts do play a powerful role in maintaining dysfunctional moods and behaviors regardless of their origins.

Emotional states, whatever their origin, carry characteristic patterns of thinking. Anxiety carries thoughts of danger and vulnerability; anger carries thoughts of violation and unfairness; paranoia carries thoughts of abuse, intrusion, persecution and frustration. As we are aware, challenges such as anxiety plague people living with an NCD on a day-to-day basis. Therapeutic change of these challenges through the application of CBT can be expedited by identification and evaluation of these thoughts.

During his training, Beck grew interested in depression and CBT. He studied how, and what, people think and concluded that depression is a distortion of the thinking process. His belief is that people think and then the feelings follow the thought. The aim of CBT is therefore to modify faulty or unproductive thinking, referred to as distorted cognition. When people are encouraged to think differently their feelings change and reality is tested to establish how the conclusions are true.

There are limitations when it comes to choosing this type of therapy. Evidence suggests that people need to be reasonably intelligent (however, this form of therapy doesn't always appeal to very intelligent people) and is ineffective for those who are deemed to be deeply disturbed. As therapy is aimed at addressing specific problems and seeking their solutions, it is not useful for personal growth. Nor is CBT believed to be useful for people with serious interpersonal or relationship difficulties.

If we think about CBT as a cognitive model, psychological disturbance is seen as a result of some malfunction in interpreting and evaluating experience, with the ultimate aim being to teach the person to monitor their thought processes and reality test them.

The reader can already see how CBT can impact positively on those experiencing negative, unhelpful thoughts and images as a result of their NCD, where a therapeutic alliance is required between therapist and client. As well as qualities such as warmth, transparency, empathy and genuineness, CBT also adds:

- *Collaboration* – The active state of working together as a team toward agreed goals. As you will recall, this fits well with Shared Action Planning, which I always use in clinical practice.

- *Guided discovery* – Which enables the client to analyze the situation and they can then draw their own conclusions.

According to Padesky (1993), guided discovery generally consists of the following:

1. A series of questions to uncover relevant information outside the client's current awareness.

2. Accurate listening and reflection by the therapist.

3. Summarizing the information discovered.

4. Synthesizing questions that ask the client to apply the new information discussed to his or her own belief.

Dr Beck has established that:

- *Automatic thoughts* flow through our mind unplanned throughout the day (words, images, memories, etc.).

- *Underlying assumptions* are beliefs or rules that guide our life. They include "should" statements and conditional "If–then" beliefs. They can guide behavior and expectations even if not in conscious awareness.

- A *schemata* is an absolutist core belief about self, others and the world. They can be positive or negative (e.g. people can't be trusted, I cannot be wrong). Schemata have been described as the screens or filters that process and code stimuli.

The three levels of thought and interconnected schema lead to underlying assumptions and these determine the type of automatic thoughts that occur. An example might be "My memory is so poor I can't even remember people's names. I will end up offending even my friends and will have a dreadful time at the party." Later in this chapter, we will consider a case study where I use CBT to address this negative thinking.

The three main goals of CBT are:

1. To relieve symptoms and resolve problems.

2. To help the individual to develop coping strategies.

3. To help the individual to modify underlying cognitive structures (beliefs and attitudes) in order to prevent relapse.

The overall strategies of CBT are:

1. To clarify the problem.

2. To describe the feelings.

3. To uncover the automatic negative thought.

4. To discover the underlying assumption (belief, attitude, value).

5. To generate an alternative thought (the therapist and client collaborate on this).

6. To reality test (homework to test new thought).

7. To give feedback (client to therapist).

The aim of collaboration:

1. Allows input from the person who knows most about the problem.

2. Encourages use of self-help techniques.

3. Encourages the client to take control of the session and reduces conflict.

The methods used in CBT to help modify negative thinking are:

1. *Reality testing* – During this experience, the client is taught to question the evidence for the automatic thought.

2. *Looking for alternatives* – This is when the client is asked for alternative explanations or solutions until as many as possible are uncovered. At the beginning these are likely to be negative before more positive and constructive thoughts develop. It removes the blinkered views that often accompany emotional rises.

3. *Reattribution* – This is where the cause of or responsibility for an event is reattributed (the client is encouraged to consider possible alternative causes for events).

4. *Decatastrophizing* – This relates to the "What if" technique.

5. *Advantages and disadvantages* – Listing these two opposites can often be a useful exercise that helps the client put things into perspective.

No matter where somebody is along their unique journey of cognitive change, they continue to have dreams, goals and aspirations. Ask yourself "Do we really ever self-actualize?" If we do, then can we achieve this state more than just the one time? In CBT, there are typical questions that we will ask to help uncover goals and to explore dreams, aspirations and desires. Reflection is not about regrets or "What if" but about what *was* achieved and what can *still* be achieved.

Such questions may be:

- If you were given three wishes what would you wish for? Why?

- If you went to bed tonight and all your problems were solved by magic, how would you know when you woke up?

- What do you want most out of life?

- Have you had treatment before? What did you gain from it?

- If you became a super hero for a day, what would you do?

- Who is your favorite sports person? What is special about them?

Let us consider how CBT can help with anxiety management. You will recall from earlier chapters the both fear and anxiety are the fuels that provide nutrition to the BPSD. Therefore, CBT can have a positive impact in reducing this fuel.

There are many anxiety disorders, and in the previous chapter I demonstrated how NLP was used to help Caroline manage her severe panic attacks, decreasing them by a significant amount. Other anxiety disorders include phobias, post-traumatic stress disorder and obsessive compulsive behavior disorder. Cognitive components of anxiety include the perception of danger, vulnerability or threat. The thoughts often accompanying anxiety begin with the dreaded *What if?* question and contain the implication that something bad is about to happen. We saw in the case of Caroline that panic is extreme anxiety that is accompanied by catastrophic misinterpretation of body and mental sensations as impending doom or death.

This anxiety can be diminished or even extinguished completely, through cognitive reconstruction, hypno-psychotherapy, self-hypnosis and overcoming avoidance.

CASE STUDY

Jim is a retired marine and a very proud man. For him, having developed NCD due to Alzheimer's disease at the age of 62 (which is classified as young onset dementia) is both degrading and demeaning. On receipt of diagnosis, both his confidence and self-esteem took a huge blow.

Recently Jim was invited to a reunion of retired marines, and he was initially excited. Anxiety then began to take over due to the core belief that his memory was no longer working. He made the following statement to his wife: "My memory is so poor I can't even remember people's names. I will end up offending even my friends and will have a dreadful time at the party."

In Figure 8.1, you will see a thought record sheet that is often used during CBT. Very often, I will encourage the client to complete this whenever needed. However, in this case, I worked intensely with Jim to change his thinking as the reunion was only 3 days away.

You will see it is separated into six columns, and there are questions that I was able to work through with Jim for each of them.

Table 8.1 Thought record sheet for Jim

Situation	Emotions/moods (rate 0–100%)	Physical sensations	Unhelpful thoughts/ images	Alternative/realistic thought	What I did/what I could do/defusion technique/what's the best response re-rate emotion 1–100%

Questions Asked of Jim

Situation

Describe what happened, where you were, when it was, who you were with and how the situation arose.

Response

I was looking at the invitation and my wife told me I had looked at it 20 times already and that nothing had changed on it since the last time 2 minutes ago! It was about 10am yesterday in the dining room and she was very harsh, impatient even, which is so unlike Amanda.

Emotions/moods (rate 0–100%)

What emotion did you feel at that time? What else was going on? How intense was it?

Response

I felt hurt when she said that. Then I thought to myself: "My memory is so poor I can't even remember people's names. I will end up offending even my friends and will have a dreadful time at the party." I was trying to remember the name of my sergeant, but I couldn't and I was his major. I always liked him, had a lot of respect for him but I just couldn't remember his bloody name. My internal wounding was about 85 percent.

Physical sensations

What did you notice in your body? Where did you feel it?

Response

I started swinging back and forth in my chair, wringing my hands. I could feel I was getting agitated.

Unhelpful thoughts/images

What went through your mind? What disturbed you? What did those thoughts/images/memories mean to you, or say about the situation? What are you responding to? What button is being pressed? What would be the worst thing about that, or that could happen?

Response
I felt belittled. I thought to myself "Why does she treat me like this?" I was, and am, responding to something that might be true. What if *(and there you have the "What if" scenario)* I am losing my mind? Going crazy?

Alternative/realistic thought
Stop and take a breath. Is this fact or opinion? What would someone else say about this situation? What's the bigger picture? Is there another way of seeing it? What advice would you give to someone else? Is your reaction in proportion to the actual event? Is this really as important as it seems?

Response
Well, it's fact that I have dementia so it's fact that my memory is really bad! My best friend would say, "So, you think memory is everything? That you've gone through your entire life never forgetting anything? What about that time when you forgot to pick me up from the barracks – left me there, stranded." He always tells me about that night [He giggled. I smiled. We laughed about this together]. I would probably tell them not to worry about it; that there are far more important things to think about. I guess being forgetful isn't such a big deal after all; I mean, I may not remember their names but they will certainly remember mine! [At that point he winked at me – after all, he did retire with the rank of major].

What I did/what I could do/defusion technique/what is the best response? (re-rate emotion 0–100%)
What could you do differently? What would be more effective? Do what works and act wisely! What would be most helpful for you or the situation? What will the consequences be?

This final column and questions is where Jim needed coaching and support. We explored the things he could do differently, and the responses he could make. He did have a sense of humor that came out in bundles once the therapeutic alliance was established and developed. Therefore, I guided him in that general direction in order to bring that part of his personality into play as we worked toward modifying negative thinking.

First, I encouraged Jim to reality test the available evidence for his automatic thought. He concluded that it was his own response that led to him feeling the way he did. We did some memory testing and the outcomes demonstrated that his memory wasn't all that poor after all! This encouraged him to realize that the ABC rules (activating event, belief system and consequence) had emerged and that his own belief had led to his actual response to his wife's comment. As we saw in NLP, if you don't like a behavior or belief, change it.

I then guided Jim into seeking positive alternatives. This was what he presented:

- My wife, and everyone else, has an opinion.

- People are entitled to express their thoughts.

- I have my own opinions and express them at will.

- I have built a shield around me – anyone's negativity directed at me will rebound back onto them.

This we made into an aide memoire card, which he kept in his pocket and also pinned a copy on the fridge door.

Moving on to the reattribution stage Jim had already recognized that his wife was experiencing stressful situations and having difficulty dealing with his diagnosis. They had discussed counseling and she had arranged an appointment to see a therapist within the next few weeks. Not only are we using CBT at this point, but the Dementia Triangle and model of psycho-social support are being used as reference and guidance tools.

Next we considered the decastrophizing element of the process where the "What if?" question is addressed. The aim in Jim's case was to get him thinking in terms of "What if I remember my sergeant's name?" "What if I remember the names of other people?" "What if I don't remember their names?" I encouraged him to think about the worst that could happen if he wasn't able to recall someone's name. The conclusion was "Well, all I need to do is ask them – and even then, it's not an issue if I forget it again."

We ended the session with Jim taking a sheet of paper and drawing a line down the middle. On the left he wrote "Advantages" and "Disadvantages" of thinking and reacting differently. He was astonished to see the column relating to advantages filled up a lot quicker than the alternative column.

CBT had a positive impact on both Jim and Amanda, and he attended the reunion, had a great time and even met some new friends. One of those new friends had also recently been diagnosed with NCD due to Alzheimer's disease, which provided Jim another level of support and comradeship.

Chapter 9

Interventions That Positively Support People Who Have an NCD and Who Also Have an Autistic Disorder

Autism is a lifelong condition. A UK government survey in 2015 suggests that 1 in 45 children, ages 3 to 17, have been diagnosed with autism spectrum disorder (ASD) (Zablotsky et al. 2015). In America, the Centers for Disease Control and Prevention (CDC) estimate that 1 in 68 children have been diagnosed.

Statistically speaking, the prevalence rates are unclear; however, we know that boys and men are over five times more likely to be diagnosed than girls. My 24-year-old daughter is one of the girls diagnosed when she was approximately 4 years old. Fortunately for her, it was an area that I specialized in prior to her birth, thus I was able to ensure she was assessed and diagnosed without delay. We are not clear whether people who have an autistic disorder (AD) are at a greater risk of developing an NCD or whether it acts as a buffer to reduce the risk. What is clear is that people with certain forms of AD have a longevity that is not different to those deemed not to have an AD; thus, they may or may not develop an NCD in later life.

The free dictionary by Farlex defines autism as a complex developmental disorder distinguished by difficulties with social interaction, verbal and non-verbal communication and behavior problems including repetitive behaviors and narrow focus of interest. There are four different types of ASDs. They are classic (or Kanner syndrome), Asperger's syndrome, pervasive development disorder not otherwise specified (PDD-NOS) or atypical autism and childhood disintegrative disorder.

For the purposes of this chapter, I am going to focus my attention on adults who have been diagnosed as living with an AD. As you will see from Figure 9.1, the triad of impairments, there is a great deal of similarity to the challenges faced by people living with an NCD and if a person with an AD does develop one of the primary NCDs, clinicians are already equipped with skills and techniques to help from a therapy or treatment point of view. Social communication, social interaction and social imagination often present as day-to-day challenges to those living through cognitive change.

Currently, we do not have enough clinical evidence to show that autism and dementia are linked. Nor do we know how many people are currently living with co-morbidity. There may be genetic similarities, but again more research is needed before we can draw any conclusions.

Previous chapters discussed the use of various therapies including CBT, hypno-psychotherapy and NLP. Now I consider whether these modalities are useful in improving the quality of life of people living with an NCD who also have a diagnosis that places them on the autism spectrum, and other strategies that can achieve a state of well-being. First, let's consider the triad of impairments and how they relate to each journey.

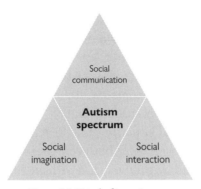

Figure 9.1 Triad of impairments

Social communication relates to challenges with communication, both verbal and non-verbal, with many people living with an AD having a literal understanding of language. An example would be going to the pub and buying a pint. If the landlord was to say "This is on the house," the person with an AD would likely take it literally. Body language, which we all rely on, may be totally alien to those with autism. Challenges that present may be things like:

- Difficulties in understanding jokes.

- Difficulties understanding sarcasm.

- Unusual and inappropriate tone of voice.

- Difficulty differentiating nouns and pronouns.

- Echolalia.

Challenges with social communication differ greatly between those with true autism, or Kanner syndrome, and those with high functioning autism, or Asperger's syndrome. If we were to correlate this with people living with an NCD, we see some similarities, again, dependent on the type of NCD and their location within their journey. People with an NCD may have reached that point in a different way but nevertheless have reached that point. We have no real understanding as to whether someone with an AD who goes on to develop an NCD has more intense challenges with social communication or not.

Social interaction relates to such things as finding chatting difficult, taking what people say literally, not understanding other people's personal space or "bubble" and struggling with group activities and situations and developing friendships. Again, we see correlation between these challenges and those often faced by people living with an NCD.

Social imagination is a very ambiguous aspect of the triad of impairments, especially in those who have high functioning autism. My daughter is a prolific artist and spends most of her day writing and drawing, thus she does have an imagination. However, the challenge comes through a lack of being able to imagine alternative outcomes and living in an unpredictable world. You will recognize this as being a challenge faced by many people experiencing their unique journey through cognitive change.

I would like us to take the view that people who have lived their entire lives on the autism spectrum have developed certain coping skills and strategies that have helped them to survive in a world that is full of unpredictability; a world where they are seen as different by mainstream society. Additionally, they have spent many years experiencing the challenges faced by people who have not been placed on the autism spectrum and who develop an NCD later in life (and just for the record, as a clinician, I believe each and every one of us could be placed on the autism spectrum because we all have autism to some degree, which is why, statistically, we really have no real clue about prevalence rates!).

Due to the challenges faced by those who do have co-morbidity, we must adapt both our clinical approach and the therapies we choose to help people deal with the symptoms that may diminish their very sense of being, purpose and personhood. While we can consider using CBT, NLP, hypno-psychotherapy or other modalities, it may be necessary to bring in other strategies such as mirroring (we discussed this in Chapter 7), gentle teaching, sensory integration therapy and music therapy. In this chapter I have space to examine one approach that I developed in detail: MaRTiS™, which is based around music and has been extremely effective for a number of years.

Music Therapy

As a clinical dementia specialist based in the UK during the first decade of 2000, I wanted to find an approach to care that would improve quality of life and perhaps even manage some of the BPSD. At the time, I had three patients who had both Asperger's syndrome and NCD due to Alzheimer's disease.

Knowledge of this co-morbidity among generic clinicians and specialists was very minimal and education for the general public wasn't all that great.

Care home communities were not geared up for providing a service to this client group, and training was not accessible to them.

I looked at possible options and considered Kitwood's ideals about person centered care. Dementia Care Mapping was a tool beginning to emerge and I decided it was time to do something; though at that point I was not sure what that should be.

On learning that the music center of the brain is in a different area to that of speech and language, it became obvious that music was the greatest communication tool in our armory. I therefore developed something called MaRTiS™ – Music and Reminiscence Therapy Incorporating Storytelling.

This approach has excellent therapeutic outcomes with this cohort no matter where they may be in their journey.

The following model, while basic in presentation, is extremely effective in improving quality of life for people living with AD and NCD, and those accompanying them through their unique, adventurous journeys.

We must always remember there is no greater force than the mind itself. When combined with music, the power of communication is enhanced to its greatest potential. This approach helps clinicians, and others, to deliver the best therapy possible and, in doing so, have a positive impact on their lives.

The Nightingale Model for the Application of MaRTiS™ Therapy

This model is the core of MaRTiS™. It encompasses the five facets of true person centered care as outlined below.

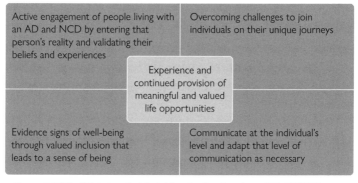

Figure 9.2 The Nightingale Model for the Application of MaRTiS Therapy

This approach is fully inclusive and puts the client at the center of any assessment, treatment or therapy, whether it is music-based or otherwise.

Experience and continued provision of meaningful and valued life opportunities

As clinicians, one of our greatest communication skills is the ability to listen. All our clients, despite age, have valued experiences they can share with us. Our approach, and therapeutic relationship, depends heavily on our acceptance and knowledge of the client's past experiences. One of the goals during MaRTiS™ is to assist the individual to improve areas in their cognitive abilities and provide activities of daily living that will assist them to enjoy further valued life opportunities. The individual must feel a sense of empowerment and control throughout the entire therapy; a sense of safety and security. Each individual must feel confident that the clinician can be trusted unconditionally.

Active engagement of people living with an AD and NCD by entering that person's reality and validating their beliefs and experiences

We all know and accept that for the most successful outcomes the clinician must step outside of their reality and into that of the person they are supporting. I may be living in November 2018, sitting at my desk writing a book; however, Paul might be stuck in reliving a past experience that occurred in 1972 – I must enter that timeframe and embark on that aspect of the journey with him. Validation of his current beliefs and experiences strengthens his trust in me, increases his confidence to share that experience and gives me permission to assist him to find a solution that will resolve the issue. As such, trust in a group setting also evolves, leading to a more meaningful relationship with his peers.

Overcoming challenges to join individuals on their unique journeys

It may seem an obvious statement, but some people don't see that clinicians are human beings. None of us is flawless and most of us have misconceived ideas about an area of expertise prior to specialist training. We must overcome our own challenges and feel confident that we can support people in a therapeutic setting. The message to all the clinicians that I have taught over the years, those I am currently teaching and those I will teach in the future, is not to be afraid to join the journey. Climb on board and partake in whatever adventure lies ahead. We are all in it together – from the person living with an AD and NCD through to the assistant serving the individual in the store.

Evidence signs of well-being through valued inclusion that leads to a sense of being

A huge part of MaRTiS™ is about valued inclusion. The clinician does not dictate what the therapy plan is going to be. Instead, we develop this together. We do not lead the MaRTiS™ session. Instead, our role is to support the client to lead and facilitate sessions.

Communicate at the individual's level and adapt that level of communication as necessary

As we specialize in this field, it is essential to understand that verbal communication isn't as important as we sometimes think. We therefore look at it this way: throughout our entire lives, verbal communication accounts for only 27 percent of contact with each other. The remainder, a staggering 73 percent of communication, is via body language. For this reason, we do not get hung up on the fact that someone may no longer be able to communicate verbally. Indeed, there are many documented cases, and I have included such a case later in this chapter, where someone may not be able to "speak" a sentence but they can still "sing" a song.

We must fine-tune our ability to read body language. We might use mirroring techniques, that is, if someone makes facial gestures or body movements, we respond by mirroring those same movements. This helps establish a relationship and increases the chance of a positive therapeutic alliance. We may sing with the client – as mentioned above, the loss of ability to use the spoken word very often does not prevent the person from singing – this fact is due to the part of the brain responsible for music being located in a different area than that of speech and language, or the Broca's and Wernicke's areas of the brain.

The Process of MaRTiS™

MaRTiS™ is an aid to communication; an interactive therapy based on *true* person centered care.

The clinician is responsible for bringing together six people into the group situation. The six will have some things in common, though this does not have to be a huge list. It is unlikely you will have six people with both AS and an NCD in the same area, so, as I do, including even one such person in the group of six is acceptable.

> TIP
>
> Complete a Life Story Profile with each individual and highlight all common interests and themes. For example, Alice and Joan both worked in a store. Bill and Alec like Frank Sinatra. Also, note down all their musical tastes and source CDs in that genre.

The only materials you will need for a MaRTiS™ session is the CDs and a CD player. Optional are musical instruments.

Once the six have been brought together, the next stage is to identify which member of the group will lead and facilitate the session (remember, this can be a different person each week).

> **TIP**
>
> For the first session, it is advisable that the most assertive and vocal person act as lead facilitator. This way, other members of the group may feel more comfortable opting to do it in following weeks.

Sessions are to be held weekly, for a total of 6 weeks. Most sessions run for approximately 1 hour, but I have found that you learn to read when it is time to stop!

At the beginning of session 1, support the lead facilitator, who will encourage the group to introduce themselves – you may choose to do an ice breaker based on a musical topic if necessary.

> **TIP – ICE BREAKER**
>
> Chose the first verse of a popular song. Make sure it is a short verse. Take six pieces of paper and write one or two words on each piece of paper. Give one piece of paper to each member of the group. Support the lead facilitator to encourage everyone to sing a word or two of that song. If the person is unable to read the word, sing it with them. This should help people feel at ease with each other and begin communication and socialization among the group.

Time to Talk

It is now time to begin a topic of conversation. Start with some recent event that will lead in to positive, past experiences for members of the group.

> **TIP – PSYCHOLOGICAL**
>
> This is where psychology plays a role. Take the knowledge you have learned from each individual and apply it to the conversation – of course, there is no breach of confidentiality as you do not identify the individual. Cross-reference with

the topic. For example, you know that Alice worked at a huge department store for many years. "Alice, haven't department stores changed these days? I was in one the other day and they were playing some awful music. What music reminds you of department stores when you were a little younger?"

You now have a topic of conversation that everyone can join in with – the lead facilitator is ready to press the CD play button as soon as the conversation dries up, or once people begin to lose focus on the discussion.

And this is how the session runs. Discuss a topic, play some music, maybe sing a song that relates directly to the theme.

Try to remain positive. However, on occasion, a negative memory may emerge and emotions may run high.

TIP – SUPPORTING A NEGATIVE EMOTION

It is okay for someone to get upset, to cry, to get agitated or even angry. These are perfectly normal responses to situations. Remember to enter that person's reality and support them through this experience. A group hug is always a show of support. For example, Bill brings up that his wife Matilda has passed away; that he misses her greatly, especially when they used to go shopping together. Actively listen to Bill and reassure him by saying "Let's spend a few moments talking about Matilda and the fun things you did together." Through the process of spotlighting, you will identify something Bill says that will offer you an opportunity to validate his emotions and move toward another path of conversation. For example, Bill might say: "After shopping, we would go to watch a James Bond film." This is your cue: "James Bond – I love James Bond. What's your favorite all-time James Bond film?" Of course you know what it is, because this would have been identified during the Life Story work. Now you can move on to James Bond music and sing along to "Goldfinger" or a related song.

Be prepared to be caught off guard. This is where your skills will allow you to respond positively to anything that happens.

CASE STUDY

For 5 weeks I had been working with a group in a Liverpool Nursing Home. There were six members in the group, four women and two men. One of the women was called Mari, and she had both Asperger's syndrome and vascular NCD (name changed to protect and respect this individual's privacy).

Each Wednesday afternoon we would meet in the leisure room. Members of the direct care team would assist people to the room and help them get comfortable in the cozy armchairs and sofa.

Mari was the only person using a wheelchair. I had chosen her for the group because she appeared to be withdrawn into herself and each time she was made cozy on one of the armchairs she would slump down and close her eyes.

Mari was born in the Scottish Highlands in 1931 in a village called Lewiston, which is one of the villages that surrounds the infamous Loch Ness. It wasn't until she was 53 that she received a diagnosis of Asperger's syndrome. At 76 she developed vascular NCD.

This was of great interest to me as I once lived in the next village – Drumnadrochit. The view from my window was Loch Ness with Urquhart Castle in the background.

In the fifth week, Mari did her usual thing of slumping into her chair and did not participate in anything I and the group tried. I was under the impression that Mari had entered her own safe world that kept her free from any further harm.

In one last attempt to reach Mari we played a piece of Scottish Highland music. Then I brought up the topic of Loch Ness, and whatever lives in the Loch. The group began to talk about the "monster" but Mari remained slumped in her chair with her eyes firmly shut. I sighed and felt a tinge of sadness knowing that Mari was lost to this world.

Suddenly, she opened her eyes and leaned forward. Looking round at the group, then directly at me, she spoke. Mari had a soft-spoken Scottish accent – and this was the first time I had heard it.

Salmon; there are salmon in that water.

With that, Mari closed her eyes, leaned back and slumped into her usual position.

She had been deemed to be in the end stages of dementia for at least 12 months. To my mind – a young dementia specialist, green in the true ways in which dementia affects the mind, body and soul – Mari was lost. How wrong I was.

This taught me a valuable lesson: Never write anyone off; always assume that the person can hear and comprehend everything that is being said. Never *do* something to an individual; instead always do things *with* the person.

For a very brief moment Mari was alive. A spark had ignited her mind; her thoughts. She expressed a sign of well-being when I thought this could never happen.

Chapter 10

Ameliorating Transitional Shock

Transitional shock is a serious condition that has been proven to cause severe psychological and physiological effects in older people. The American term is *relocation syndrome*.

The term "transitional shock" is used throughout this chapter as any major change to a person's life could result in its manifestation – it is not confined to relocation only, although this is my main focus here.

It has been my aim to describe and define transitional shock and to suggest ways to ameliorate it, in addition to ways of minimizing the risk of it developing in any one individual. I have also included some suggested recommendations and an example of a transitional checklist.

It is my belief that every clinician and practitioner involved in the journey of those living with an NCD should have a sound knowledge of transitional shock – especially as services expand and develop on a regular basis. To have this knowledge equips professionals with the knowledge, skills and competencies to ensure each person receives the greatest quality of care available should this ever become a problem at any time during their care.

This chapter has particular relevance to all those involved in meeting holistic care needs, including doctors, nurses, social workers, managers and care assistants. In addition, students of these disciplines can also benefit from gaining an understanding of the importance of ameliorating transitional shock.

Prior to getting involved in this area of interest, I surveyed a number of clinicians and practitioners from various areas within the care sector. This included both statutory and non-statutory bodies. In total, 100 individual professionals completed the questionnaire, with the following results (see also Appendix 1):

- 75 percent of respondents had never heard of transitional shock.

- 18 percent of respondents had heard of transitional shock but had no knowledge of it.

- 7 percent of respondents had heard of transitional shock and felt they had the necessary knowledge, skills and competencies to deal with it if it was presented by their present client group.

What Is Transitional Shock?

Transitional shock may be triggered by change, either in the living environment or way of life, and may lead to individuals experiencing very serious negative physiological and psychological disorders (Ivanis 1992).

Much academia has been dedicated to loss and bereavement, which, in essence, may be contributors to the development of transitional shock as individuals experience a huge sense of loss.

In her book *Living through Personal Crisis*, Ann Kaiser Stearns (1984) writes "To the ancient Egyptians the phoenix was a legendary bird, consumed by fire, who rose up from its own ashes and assumed a new life. From our own ashes we also must recreate ourselves, our lives." For the majority of those living with an NCD, which includes those who are being supported in long-term residential, nursing or memory care environments, some, or all, aspects of their life are constantly being recreated. For this reason, support and excellent planning are required to ensure the transition is successful for each person and to minimize the possibilities of transitional shock manifesting at any time before, during or even after the change.

Moving home is a stressful event in anyone's life. The vast array of emotional effects of stress can vary but may include both verbal and physical aggression directed at the individual themselves or toward those supporting the journey. A person may become more active, more irritable, critical, fearful and anxious. A further form of response is withdrawal, self-criticism and reduction in activity. If we consider the implications of this level of unsafe stress, it is easy to comprehend the difficulties that may present.

Extreme responses to relocation have been observed among elderly people, people with an NCD of all ages, people with intellectual disabilities and those with enduring mental health challenges, including some who may become profoundly depressed, refuse to eat, lose weight and weep a great deal. Transitional shock may not appear immediately. A person may look as though he or she has settled in well but after several weeks, or even months, show signs that something may be wrong. All staff should therefore be alert to the long-term effects of relocation.

People being supported in long-term care settings have often been moved around with total disregard for their feelings and with no, or very little, preparation. Impersonal organizations have lifted them out of one setting and dropped them into another. It is highly likely that such inconsiderate and poor management has been a direct cause of some of their emotional and physical problems, which have then been wrongly attributed to their age, NCD or other individual problem.

From the evidence documented above, I define transitional shock as:

> A process whereby an individual experiences negative and undesirable change of physical and psychological effects due to a sudden change of environment or way of life without receiving adequate support prior, during and after the change has occurred.

One example of this is when an individual moves from one long-term living environment, such as a residential home (where he or she has lived in a safe, secure environment for many years) into a nursing home without adequate support and planning from the responsible services.

Accepted practice is now to ensure a gradual transition period is observed through a well-prepared care package. However, it must be accepted that this is not always possible in services that provide memory care. At times such as during an emergency or crisis when immediate intervention is necessary (and when necessary interventions cannot be provided in place, which should always be the first-line choice), gradual transition is not an option.

We can go a long way to preventing such immediate relocation through adequate in-place provision.

What Are Some Effects of Transitional Shock?

This will inevitably vary from one individual to the other and range from mild to severe. Some effects have been identified above but evidence from studies shows that women and those with a severe cognitive impairment or change experience far more severe effects than people with no known impairment, or a mild to moderate cognitive change (Ivanis 1992). Signs may manifest at any time. However, some effects are shown to be presented by a high proportion of those experiencing the effects of transitional shock.

These can be divided into two categories, although some may fall into both:

Psychological

- Verbal/physical aggression
- Self-injurious behavior
- Inexplicable weeping
- Mood swings
- Withdrawal
- Depression
- Lethargy

Physiological

- Various physical illnesses in elderly men
- Increased appetite/weight gain
- Decreased appetite/weight loss
- Disturbed sleep
- Constipation
- Incontinence
- Headache
- Diarrhea

Steps to Take to Ameliorate Transitional Shock

Every individual living with an NCD should have a care package that includes a plan concerning preparation for their future residential provision. This should include ways of adapting to being separated from family, close friends and past staff members who have supported the individual most closely. Some or all of the tools and models discussed so far throughout this book are likely to be of use here.

Ideally, both aging in place and supporting someone living with an NCD in place is preferable to relocation. However, this isn't always possible, hence the need for such communities as memory care and nursing homes. Visits to any potential new home should be for short periods of time to begin with, and in a different environment with different people, such as short-term care. If the individual is introduced to the future change through short visits and stays, then when the time comes for a longer-term change, he or she is far more likely to adapt more positively.

Relocation (of any kind) should not be forced on people. Help and support must be offered in an attempt to help individuals decide for themselves. As a clinician I place a great emphasis on empowerment and true person centered care. However, empowerment in this way is not always an option, as in the case of a move being necessary to facilitate an emergency service change, but choices of where a person goes to live, and with whom, can still be offered. Individuals have the right to make these choices, to participate and to contribute as much as they are able to do so in their own transition.

If the individual wishes, close relatives, friends and advocates should also be involved as much as possible before, during and after the change.

Since relocation can prove stressful, attempts should be made to avoid other stresses at the same time. For example, changing from one daytime occupation or activity to another at the same time as moving to a new living environment makes two major transitions, which would be better spread over a specified period of time.

Discussions of every aspect of the transition beforehand could prove very beneficial. Individuals should have the chance to say how they feel. They may have fears and concerns, which can be dealt with if they are brought to light. Alternatively, they may be unduly optimistic, thus increasing the possibility that their expectations will be dashed. A realistic appraisal of events is likely to assist adjustment. Always remember to work with the person's reality as it may well be different to yours. As we know, validation can assist the person a great deal.

Preliminary visits to the new living environment should always be part of the transitional plan. These visits should be enjoyable and increased in length at each visit. A friendly, informal and relaxed atmosphere will help the person feel much more at ease and less anxious.

In any transition there is likely to be some form of loss and the greater the loss, the greater the emotional upset. Therefore, a reduction in personal losses by maintaining as much continuity as possible must be set as an initial goal.

TIP

This can be done by ensuring that personal possessions move with the individual, thus acting as an anchor to that particular person. Daily routines should not be so radically different to begin with. Any necessary changes to routine ought to be initiated prior to the move if this is possible, thus allowing the person to adjust to the new routine in the old, familiar environment.

Prophylactic Measures to Prevent Manifestations of Transitional Shock

There are three stages that present the risk of transitional shock developing and manifesting. These stages are:

Stage 1 pre-transition

Stage 2 transition

Stage 3 post-transition

Pre-transition

The most important factor at this stage is adequate planning with full involvement of the individual concerned at all times and during all decision making processes (full involvement refers to the individual contributing as much as he or she is able). Service providers, clinicians and practitioners must work together with the person to ensure he or she is fully aware of all developments and/or setbacks influencing the transition. Each member of the multidisciplinary team must take equal and joint responsibility to minimize the risks. There must always be an adequate transition period to help the individual accept the transition prior to it taking place. An appropriate checklist/monitoring system should be in place at this stage, to monitor and record things that concern the individual about the change; for example, he or she may be concerned about losing contact with a certain person. Action must be taken to help alleviate these concerns by the appropriately skilled clinician, who can record and document their input as well as appraise the multidisciplinary team in order to keep them updated about the situation and further proactive intervention that may be indicated.

Transition

There must be an adequate support network established, and in place, by the time the transition occurs. This may include having appointed a member of the direct care team as the individual's transition worker; having an appropriate monitoring system in his/her personal file; having an intervention strategy in place should it be required; and ensuring the individual, family members, friends and advocates are fully aware of the clinical support available to them as long as it is needed by the person(s).

Post-transition

At this stage the individual must be allowed the opportunity to maintain contact with people he or she has moved away from. These may be life partners and other family members, friends, caregivers, etc., and this can be done via visits, telephone conversations or letter – the transition worker co-coordinating this along with the individual. He or she must be encouraged to express his or her own positive, and also negative, feelings about the change and to discuss advantages and disadvantages. Counseling will inevitably help the person to adapt and accept the change more readily. Again, there must be an appropriate monitoring system and intervention strategy in place with the transition worker continuing to support when necessary.

Access to other professionals must be made available at all times and referrals made where and when necessary.

Relation of Theory to Practice
Scenario Based on a Factual Case

Turner House is both a rehabilitation residential and nursing home for people who live with rare forms of NCD and who have associated psychiatric disorders. For those people who come to reside at Turner House, a wide range of changes are experienced by them. These are both personal and environmental. For this reason, an effective management strategy is a necessity in order to maximize each individual's successful rehabilitation.

Personal changes

These include moving away from friends, family and others who have supported them for many years (this in itself can cause an individual to grieve). There is a reduction in opportunities in accordance with O'Brien's Accomplishments; expectations (from team members) of higher independence and empowerment over their own lives; acceptance of, and agreement with, certain "in-house" policies and procedures, for example, smoking policy; commitment to a possible behavior contract; and an adjustment to a sense of loss for their previous living environment and people they were/are close to.

Environmental changes

These include a complete change of home; a new team of caregivers; a new coordinator and key worker; new housemates; a different geographical location; a change to daytime occupation and routine in lifestyle; a possible change of sleeping arrangements as each person has their own room at Turner House.

Management strategy

I was the senior responsible clinician at Turner House with, among other responsibilities, a leadership role. As a team, we designed a new management strategy that proved effective in reducing the risk of development of post-transitional shock. There was also a system *in situ* for use at the pre-transitional and transitional phases of relocation of any of the individuals for when they were ready to move into a more mainstream memory care community. However, I will describe the system in use at the post-transitional stage as this relates to someone who moved to Turner House.

Post-transitional management

A 57-year-old male, M, with frontotemporal lobe NCD, severe behavioral challenges and self-injurious behavior arrived at Turner House from an acute admission/assessment ward of the local psychiatric hospital. There was very little done in the way of planning the transition and the move appeared to the team to be for political reasons. Though he did visit Turner House for a number of short stays and had some time to build the foundations of a relationship with his new coordinator, many of the resource issues were inadequately addressed and in place prior to the permanent transition. Due to the inadequate planning, the post-transitional management system was very useful, not only for the team, but also for the individual concerned.

First, M had a good relationship with his life partner and saw her regularly. Therefore, it was a necessity to maintain that relationship link – this was facilitated by his coordinator. M saw his partner whenever he wished; she had the option of staying overnight (this she did twice a week) and he spoke with her regularly via the telephone. This proved an important anchor for both M and his partner.

Second, there was a resource implication in that M required a full, structured, activity-based lifestyle. He told the team "I like to keep busy." This approach would meet the individual's own choice, assist in the management of his experiential problem behaviors and enhance his rehabilitative development. However, the implication was that the transition occurred prior to the activities being available, planned and structured. The issue was overcome through the identification of required resources, which were then provided by the necessary and relevant agencies, which included intense therapy from the psychology and psychiatry teams. A structured timetable was then designed with M. Again, the team discovered this was a vital component in contributing to a successful transition.

Third, M was given the opportunity to discuss and express his own positive and negative feelings about the change and to discuss the advantages and disadvantages.

Finally, a transitional checklist was designed and completed with M and his partner. This was a short questionnaire completed at the end of M's first month. There were 12 questions in total:

1. How many times have you moved in the last 12 months?

2. Do you live with epilepsy? An auditory problem? A visual problem? A physical disability? A psychiatric disorder?

3. Do you experience behavior which you, and/or your partner see as problematic or challenging?

4. If yes to question 3, is this aggression aimed at others? Is the aggression aimed at property? Harming yourself? Other?

5. How many times have you expressed these behaviors in the past month?

6. If you take "prn/as required medicine" to help you control these behaviors, how often have you taken it in the last month?

7. Have you been incontinent in the last month? If so, how often? Is this during the day/night/both?

8. How many times have you been ill in the last month?

9. How many accidents have you had in the last month?

10. Is your sleep: Good? Average? Disturbed?

11. What are your daytime activities?

12. Please circle the words which best describe how you have felt over the last month: happy/unhappy;

calm/agitated; has there been less problem behavior/ more problem behavior; sociable/unsociable; responsive/tired; good tempered/irritable.

The above checklist was based around M by using the Health Career Model (an assessment tool that gives a holistic assessment of an individual (King 1981)). The choice of language used was based around M's own understanding of certain words. In this example, the data were recorded at the end of the first month and an identical questionnaire would be completed each month for a total of 6 months. By analyzing the data on a monthly basis, in conjunction with the completed daily report, any changes in physical and/or psychological health could be identified; therefore, allowing rapid and effective intervention whenever necessary.

Postscript

It is appropriate to state that any negative changes to a person's physical or psychological health indicated by the data are not fully conclusive that he or she is experiencing transitional shock.

It is at this stage that a multidisciplinary team meeting is required in order for all options to be explored and a decisive conclusion or clinical diagnosis reached and acted on.

Conclusion

Transitional shock is caused by inadequate planning prior, during and after a major change has occurred to an individual's life. A number of stress-related disorders may be experienced, exacerbated by those two fuels, fear and anxiety.

Major change is a difficult issue for most people and when you add to the mix additional cognitive change and psychiatric disorders, these difficulties are intensified.

Recommendations

The following recommendations are aimed at reducing the risk of transitional shock occurring in those who may face major changes to their life on a regular basis. Where transitional shock does manifest these recommendations will ensure the condition is clinically managed effectively in the interests of the individual.

- That a member of the existing direct care team be appointed to act as a transition worker in each home.

- That the lead clinician (physician or consultant) be the first point of contact for all concerned about any physical effects of a transition.

- That training is made available to direct care staff, especially those acting in the role of transition worker, in order to equip them with the necessary skills needed to fulfill the role in a competent manner.

- That each service has an appropriate transition monitoring system in place for each individual facing a major life change. This system must be based on the individual concerned, taking into consideration his or her personality and character and past history; therefore, a universal system does not exist but a SAP is essential.

- That each service has an appropriate, reactive intervention strategy in place for the effective management of transitional shock should it occur.

APPENDIX 1 QUESTIONNAIRE

Please answer the following questions with accuracy and honesty.

1. Have you ever heard of the term *transitional shock*?

2. Do you have any knowledge of transitional shock?

3. Can you briefly define transitional shock?

4. What do you think may contribute to transitional shock?

5. Would you be able to recognize the possible presence of transitional shock in those you support?

6. Would you know how to manage it should it manifest in any of the people you support?

7. Would you like to know more about transitional shock and its effects on older people, those with learning disabilities and/or mental health problems?

Those who completed the questionnaire included a cross-section of clinicians from dementia care services, learning disability services, community and ward-based psychiatric nurses, forensic psychiatrists and community psychiatric nurses, support, care and nursing assistants supporting people living with an NCD, occupational therapists, and speech and language therapists.

APPENDIX 2 TRANSITIONAL CHECKLIST

The transitional checklist is a short questionnaire that should be completed by the transition worker assigned to each person who moves into the home or community. The questionnaire is a repeated measure, being completed at the pre-transition stage, 1 month after the move and at 6 months post follow-up.

Example transitional checklist

Full name: _____

Date of birth: _____

Date of move: _____

How many times has the person moved in the last 12 months?

Please circle if the person has *epilepsy; an auditory impairment; a visual impairment; a physical impairment; a psychiatric diagnosis*

Please circle the appropriate term which would describe the person's degree of cognitive impairment: *mild; moderate; severe; profound*

Does the person have behavior described as challenging or problematic? *Yes / No*

- If yes to the preceding question, please circle the appropriate category to indicate what these problem behaviors are: *aggression to property; self-harm; other* (be specific):

  _____
  _____
  _____
  _____

How many incidents of the problem behaviors have there been during the last period? _____ incidents.

If the person is prescribed *"prn/as required medicine"* for the behaviors, how often has this been administered during the last period? _____ administrations.

Has the person been incontinent during the last period? *Yes / No*

If the person has been incontinent, how often: _____ times.

How many times has the person been ill during the last period? _____ times.

How many accident reports have been completed for this person during the last period? _____

Is the person's sleep: *good; average; disturbed.*

Please state the person's daytime activities:

_____

_____

_____

_____

Please circle the point on the scale that you think best describes how the person has been during the last period:

Happy	1 2 3 4 5 6 7	Unhappy
Calm	1 2 3 4 5 6 7	Agitated
↓ Problem behavior	1 2 3 4 5 6 7	Problem behavior ↑
Sociable	1 2 3 4 5 6 7	Unsociable
Responsive	1 2 3 4 5 6 7	Apathetic
Good tempered	1 2 3 4 5 6 7	Irritable

Any additional comments/information:

_____

_____

_____

_____

Completed by: _____ Date: ___/___/___

Use of transitional checklist

1. The transitional checklist is a useful tool for monitoring the effects of transition in anyone experiencing change. Once completed, it will show at a glance whether the person may be experiencing negative, undesirable effects.

2. This checklist is an example only and may not be suitable for each and every individual. However, it may serve as a useful guide to direct care staff wishing to design a checklist to suit individual needs.

3. Where someone has the necessary skills, he or she should always be enabled to complete the checklist along with the person responsible for its completion. This should be detailed in the SAP.

4. The completed checklists must be audited at all times, thus ensuring that direct care staff are aware of any need to design and implement the relevant intervention strategy.

5. As a shared document between professionals and others embarking on the journey of the person living with an NCD, this checklist is invaluable.

While working as part of the team that helped close Stoke Park Hospital in Bristol, UK, and relocate people into the community, this strategy was extremely valuable. Implementing individual transition management plans (ITMPs) can, and does, reduce any negative impact that change can have on those we support, and strengthens our armory as clinicians.

Chapter 11

Intensive Ranch and
Farm Retreat Therapy

I have written that communication at the appropriate level between clinician and patient/client is crucial for a positive therapeutic outcome. The CAR Approach seen in Chapter 4 further strengthens and demonstrates the point. We also explored how music, through MaRTiS™, is an excellent vehicle for tapping into memory and helping people express their emotions and feelings.

Another excellent, non-threatening mode of communication comes within the relationship one has with animals. In this chapter, through a case study, I will focus on the use of horses and goats, along with psychotherapy, as a way to help people overcome one of the serious challenges faced by those with an NCD – that of stigma.

Let's Look at Communication

Before we address the reduction of stigma through the approach of intensive ranch and farm therapy, it is important to understand the concept of communication. The *Oxford Concise English Dictionary* defines communication as "the act of imparting, especially news."

Communication is a two-way process. In psychological terms, broadly speaking, communication is the transmission of something from one location to another. The "*thing*" that is transmitted may be a message, a signal, a meaning, etc. In order to have communication both the transmitter and receiver must share a common code, so that the meaning or information contained in the message may be interpreted without error (Reber and Reber 2009). This tells us that it can be both verbal and non-verbal, thus we can maximize communication with those we support through the non-verbal language expressed by our non-human collaborators.

Clinicians supporting people living with an NCD *must* be able to facilitate communication both effectively and appropriately. Additionally, this level of communication should also extend to our colleagues, the family and friends of the people we care for and, in fact, anybody else we come into contact with. We must use all the available resources to achieve this, including the use of animal therapy.

Communication can be verbal or non-verbal. It is estimated that as much as 70 percent of human communication is carried out through non-verbal channels (Asher 1999). Through my own work in this area I estimate it to be in the region of 73 percent.

Why then do we appear to take so little notice of something that plays such a prominent part in our lives? Often, body language speaks louder than words and therefore dictates how people react to you and how you perceive them. This is especially so when we are supporting people who have an NCD to such a degree that their verbal skills are compromised and dysfunctional.

I will reiterate something I wrote previously – when supporting people along their unique journeys, make only one assumption:

> That each individual understands everything being said and all that is happening around them.

We, as clinicians, listen carefully to what the person is trying to tell us. We look at their body language and should always allow the person time to get their message across. It can take a good 30 seconds or more for somebody with a cognitive impairment to respond in a way that is appropriate to them. We must always respond to a person who is saying something because communication is behavior and therefore every behavior is a form of communication. We always explain to the person what we are going to do *before* actually doing it and we always involve the person in the decision making process. We speak clearly, whether verbal or non-verbal, using terminology that is appropriate to that person – and this may include local slang words. These are things we are taught and learn through clinical practice or family and friend interactions, yet horses do this instinctively because it is how they communicate 100 percent of the time. A few days ago I watched my herd of five horses, whose leader is a 7-year-old mustang mare called Raquel. She raised her head and glanced at each of the other four, who knew immediately what she was asking of them. The art of dressage works in the same way. There is no verbal communication between horse and rider, only very subtle body language. This mode of communication is successful with people living with an NCD, those working through post-traumatic stress disorder, individuals with learning and intellectual difficulties and many other people journeying though life's numerous challenges because there are no expectations to succeed in a goal or behave in a restricted way.

Positive interactions with those living with an NCD include respecting and valuing the individual, no matter where they are in their journey, and horses do this unconditionally. Some ways in which this is achieved include:

- Grooming – horses that are used in therapy are easy to bond with. They enjoy human contact and find grooming to be a way in which they can easily, and quickly, build a therapeutic relationship with the person using the brush on their mane, tail and body.

- Stroking – horses will come to the person to be stroked. Stroking an equine leads to a number of physiological and psychological benefits. For example, both equine and human hearts will synchronize, which helps slow down the heart rate of someone who is anxious.

- Overcoming fear – horses who feel safe and secure in their environment, and within their herds, demonstrate very little fear. This is transferred to the person, who mirrors this emotion within themselves.

- The communication systems and language – throughout our entire lives we have used body language and emotional empathy. However, it has rarely been at the conscious level. Both those living with an NCD and the clinician providing therapy/ treatment can learn to bring this to the conscious level through equine contact.

- Confidence building – learning a new skill such as the ability to ride or groom a horse is not only cathartic but gives individuals increased confidence and helps build their self-esteem.

- Preparation for intensive psychotherapy – building self-esteem and confidence through a non-threatening relationship with a horse helps equip people with sufficient emotional strength to achieve successful outcomes from any of the psychotherapeutic modalities clinicians use as part of the overall therapeutic experience.

These are just a few ways in which horse interaction plays a huge part in intensive ranch and farm retreat therapy.

Stigma was highlighted as something to be addressed in the document "Living Well With Dementia: a national dementia strategy" (DoH 2009). Stigma is a form of discrimination and stereotyping often found in all areas of mental illness, learning and intellectual disabilities and of course NCD.

Some people feel shame (as we saw with Jim in Chapter 8), which can often lead to them withdrawing from family and friends and becoming diminished due to ill-being. Stigma can also prevent individuals from achieving their set goals in therapy, and even dissuade them from entering therapy in the first place. The following scenario focuses on a lady with the early stages of young onset NCD due to Alzheimer's disease, who initially refused all offers of help, intervention and clinical support because of the shame and embarrassment she felt.

I have created the Neurocognitive Disorder Destigmatizing Model (NCD-DS Model™) for the numerous times I am faced with this issue in a clinical setting and use it to demonstrate its value with this particular lady. You can see this model in Figure 11.1.

Delivery of diagnosis must be done in a sensitive manner. Obvious statement, right? However, this is not always the case. The person should be encouraged to take someone with them when they go to see the clinician for their diagnosis. Additionally, they must ensure they have thought about any questions they wish to ask ahead of the appointment. The patient or person accompanying them should take paper and a pen so they can document what they are being told. Unfortunately, when receiving a diagnosis relating to an NCD, the patient rarely takes everything in and the clinician must be prepared to repeat themselves or use less clinical terminology.

Denial and rejection is a very common response to receiving a diagnosis such as NCD due to Alzheimer's disease. It makes sense that another appointment is scheduled by the clinician to see the patient in a few weeks' time to revisit and review the situation. I have asked many patients the following question: "Upon receiving your diagnosis, was it useful to receive all the information about what happens next at that time?" A huge majority of patients tell me that they would prefer a follow-up appointment to go through it all after about 3–4 weeks, something that makes a great deal of sense.

Clinical explanation must be done in a way that the patient can comprehend. Not too long ago I saw a patient whose neurologist had coldly told him "You have Alzheimer's. All I can do is give you a pill. You'll just deteriorate over time until you eventually die." Now, I would encourage readers of this book to think long and hard about that, and the devastating impact it had on that gentleman. As we know, there is much that can be done to address the symptoms of this disease, and those options must always be part of the clinical explanation of both diagnosis and prognosis.

The individual should be engaged by clinicians and those supporting them in order to express their emotions. These are likely to be negative, with the patient being angry, hurt, upset, confused and placed on an emotional rollercoaster. It is never acceptable to tell a patient "not to worry" or "it will be okay." It is always acceptable to enable them to express exactly how they feel – and this is the case throughout the patient's entire journey.

Empowerment is crucial. By empowering the patient to take control of the disease, the clinician makes them the key operator of their journey through cognitive change.

Ownership of the journey by the person living with an NCD is the key to destigmatizing their disease and placing it where it belongs – as part of who they are and not who they have, or will, become. I once had a patient who called his NCD his "unwanted guest" and he often told that guest just what he thought of him and that he would be evicting him anytime soon.

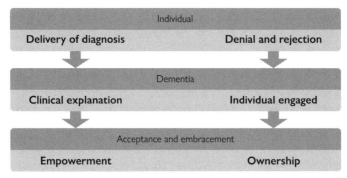

Figure 11.1 The NCD-DS Model™

CASE STUDY

Hannah is very well known and respected in the village where she has lived all her life. She does a great deal of voluntary work within the community and is always the first to step forward when a fund raising event is required. At the age of 42, she began to have difficulties with her memory. She then noticed she was getting lost on her drive to work, a route she had taken for over 7 years. Her husband knew there must be something wrong and persuaded Hannah to visit the local GP, Dr Amanda Bryce. Dr Bryce did the usual screening tests and was concerned enough to refer her to the memory clinic for a full, and more comprehensive evaluation.

After a few weeks of physical and psychological tests and scans, Hannah was given the diagnosis that she was in the early stages of young onset NCD due to Alzheimer's disease. She was absolutely broken and felt that her entire world was beginning to collapse around her. She not only felt helpless to stop what was happening to her, but she also felt stupid and ashamed. She had always been very strong and independent and had always enjoyed her roles as part-time primary school teacher and part-time community volunteer. On receiving her diagnosis Hannah just wanted to shut herself away. She refused to go out or to see anyone. She was experiencing what she referred to as a process of living bereavement.

Her husband, Alan, also felt frustrated and held the belief that "it just isn't fair." He was the village policeman, slightly older than Hannah and equally well respected by the community. He wanted to help his wife in any way he could, but she closed herself off to him too.

After 2 weeks of getting nowhere with her patient, I received the referral from Dr Bryce and went out to visit with Hannah and her husband. Though Hannah was resistant to seeing me, Alan persuaded her to at least meet me and see what I had to say. From my conversation with Alan, I could see their relationship was under a great deal of strain, his wife was angry toward everyone and everything, and he had no idea how he could support her at this time without help.

It was apparent that Hannah was very angry, and her emotions were being fueled by the usual fear and anxiety. Through the process of spotlighting, it became very clear that stigma was affecting her to a degree even I hadn't witnessed before.

As you can see in Figure 11.2, stigma was consuming Hannah's very being. It was robbing her of her confidence and self-esteem, affecting her marriage and relationship with the community she was so close to. Every aspect of her life appeared to be negative and she had closed herself off from those she knew, trusted, respected and loved.

Her belief that this living bereavement was controlling all her emotions was leading to a negative mindset, and if that mindset wasn't changed by addressing her current thinking she would not be able to pull herself out of the quagmire in which she had found herself.

She said she needed to escape: that she felt trapped in her world and that she couldn't cope with all the demands being made on her by Alan, her family and friends, her work colleagues and members of the community as a whole. Due to where she was emotionally, Hannah was unable to see that all they wanted to do was help and support her. I offered her an opportunity to visit the farm as a temporary escape, and for the first time in what Alan described as an eternity, her frown went away and she smiled. Fortunately, that smile didn't melt when I spoke to her about intensive therapy, and that Raquel, our lead mare, was an excellent therapist!

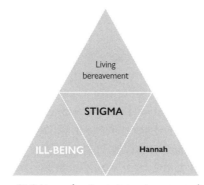

Figure 11.2 Hannah prior to intensive retreat therapy

Stigma

As you can see, stigma was leading Hannah on a very dangerous journey. The shame, guilt and helplessness that she felt were infecting the very core of her being. They had to be confronted and eliminated.

Living bereavement

Hannah was on an emotional rollercoaster when I first went to see her. She appeared to be experiencing shock, anger and denial as a combined reaction to her diagnosis, with no sign of acceptance or coping because fear and anxiety was oppressing those two positive behaviors.

Ill-being

When I met Hannah she looked thin, disheveled and unkempt. She didn't smile and her eyes were so dull I could see the sadness that was running through her entire mind, body and soul. According to Alan, this was the opposite of how she used to be. I found no signs of well-being at the start of our consultation.

Hannah

Where is Hannah, the person, the character, through all of this? I found her shriveling up and dying in the corner where stigma, and its main collaborator ill-being, wanted her to be. Her mindset was negative. Her new world was so dark she was unable to see anything good inside it and all she wanted to do was hide away from the world. I felt sure that intensive therapy over a weekend at the farm would help her to rediscover the true Hannah.

When Hannah arrived at the farm on the Friday evening, she was accompanied by Alan. However, she wanted to spend the weekend alone so her husband returned to their village, which was only 30 miles (48 km) away.

Together, through a SAP approach we agreed on the following therapy plan, which can be seen in Figure 11.3.

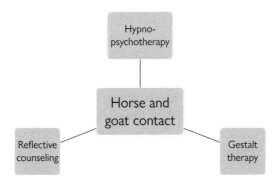

Figure 11.3 Agreed therapy plan

Horse and goat contact

This is where therapy always begins. Following breakfast, Hannah was introduced to the horses and goats and given a few hours to just "be" with them. There are no goals, no pressure, simply freedom to enjoy the space, the peace and quiet, and of course to reduce Hannah's fear and anxiety through synchronization of heart beats. The goats are very playful, and mischievous, which made Hannah laugh, therefore releasing much-needed endorphins. They enjoy being stroked and brushed and will allow someone to do this to them all day long, again assisting Hannah's brain to release some happy chemicals including serotonin, prolactin and oxytocin.

For me, this process is an adjunct to human therapy and in this case we had settled on an eclectic approach of hypno-psychotherapy, reflective counseling and Gestalt therapy. As we have already established, the ultimate goal was for Hannah to let go of all the negativity, eliminate stigma and rediscover the Hannah that once was. As clinicians we are familiar with these therapies so I will discuss the outcomes and impacts they had on Hannah as the weekend unfolded.

Hypno-psychotherapy

This modality was chosen so that I could help Hannah swiftly work through her emotional rollercoaster and let go of negative thoughts, images, experiences, beliefs and of course any negative energy that had accumulated in her mind, body and soul since receiving her diagnosis. I was also able to teach her how to do her own self-hypnosis whenever she needed to manage her inner fear and anxiety so she could remain in control of that fuel. I also incorporated both regression therapy and time lining into the four 1-hour sessions we did of this. I used the CRC Approach (Calmness and Relaxation = Confidence) to assist Hannah with regrowth of her own inner strength, confidence and self-esteem with ego-strengthening techniques used as the foundation upon which other techniques could be built. For Hannah, this improved her clarity of thinking and removed much of the pettifogging that had accumulated since the diagnosis.

Reflective counseling

For the benefit of non-therapists and non-clinicians reading this book, reflective counseling is a useful tool to help the therapist or clinician accurately evaluate the client's emotional well-being (or ill-being) by reading either verbal or non-verbal signals and messages. In order for this to be successful it is essential to actively listen, spotlight and respond to whatever the client is feeling. It's a form of empathy in that the therapist or clinician can sense the world just as the client perceives it. This was useful in addressing Hannah's belief system in terms of embarrassment and shame, and helping her to find solutions to change that belief system and her own mindset.

Gestalt therapy

I used "empty chair" therapy where Hannah created an image of Mr Stigma, who was sitting in a chair opposite where she was sitting. I encouraged her to form in her mind exactly how he looked, how he dressed and how he spoke, including his accent. After giving Hannah a few acting tips for expressing how she was feeling and also how to assertively tell Mr Stigma he was no longer going to make her feel that way, I left her to act out the scenario. She fed back how she told him that he had made her life hell but that she was now back in charge after realizing he was nothing but a sycophant who is now out of work. Her session lasted 40 minutes and when she appeared from the room she looked like a completely different person. She was calm and relaxed and appeared to be back in control. However, she said she wanted to do that one more time before the weekend was over, so this exercise constituted her final part of the therapy on Sunday evening.

Between sessions of human therapy, Hannah spent time with the horses and goats where the communication and relationship between them were non-conditional. She didn't have pets due to her busy lifestyle but, on realizing how beneficial one would be at this point in her life, and after being exposed to the farm dogs and cats, she decided she was going to get herself a cat – and that Alan would have no say in the matter. It was at that moment I knew that the intensive therapy weekend had been very successful and that the partnership between human and animal had indeed been cathartic, healing and all round therapeutic.

So what were the actual outcomes from the retreat weekend and how had it influenced positive change for Hannah? I will discuss this below by referring to Figure 11.4.

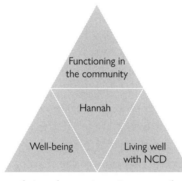

Figure 11.4 Hannah 4 weeks post-intensive retreat therapy at follow-up

Hannah is now in a much better place. Through intensive therapy she has rediscovered herself, rebuilt her confidence and self-esteem, and is once again empowered to take control of her life. No longer does she feel shame or embarrassment as the stigma is no longer present: the aim of eliminating this negative emotion was achieved.

Well-being improved immensely, not only for Hannah but her husband too. Their relationship was back on track and they were once again heading toward the strong partnership they once had. Hannah was smiling more, was more motivated and her mindset was much more positive. I had recorded the hypno-psychotherapy sessions I did with her and she had been listening to them twice a week as prescribed. Additionally, she had mastered the art of self-hypnosis and taught it to Alan so they could do it together. She had been to both her hairdresser and manicurist and was back to looking smart and professional. Even though she had decided to leave her job as a teacher due to increasing dysfunction of her immediate memory, she was positive that it had been the right decision for her. She kept a diary and a note jogger outlining her daily tasks. She pinned this to the refrigerator, which was in clear sight every time she entered the kitchen. She stated that she felt as though she had worked through the initial stages of living bereavement and that she was now at the stages of acceptance and coping, which was a major shift in such a short space of time. She still has her "blue" moments but when this happens she is supported by her husband to use the tools she developed during the intensive weekend. One final positive was that she had got herself a lap cat from the local rescue shelter, which was helping with the continued theme of animal therapy.

Living well with NCD is something we, as clinicians, aim to achieve through every stage of the journey. With the appropriate tools and change of mindset, Hannah appears to be living much better with her day-to-day challenges in many ways. We have seen a number of them while discussing her current state of well-being. The very fact that she now feels more in control of her life, and is able to think much more clearly, has resulted in both her confidence and self-esteem improving massively. With continued support from her husband, family and friends, she will find her journey much smoother despite the challenges each stage will present to them.

Functioning in the community is what maintains Hannah's motivation, purpose and meaning in life. Her input into community and events had increased since leaving her teaching post and at my follow-up she was fund raising for the local youth club. They required a new minibus and this project was now her main priority.

At the time of writing, Hannah continues to travel through her journey and has had two more weekend retreats that have taught her new tools and strategies that are helping her through the moderate stages of her cognitive change. Her case demonstrates the potential that intensive therapy can play in improving quality of life and assisting people to live as well as they can. It also demonstrates the powerful relationship between humans and non-humans and how that too can help with an individual's journey.

Chapter 12

Clinical Interventions for Adults and Children Living with Rare and Unusual Forms of Neurocognitive Disorders

The more rare and unusual forms of NCD get very little attention, but their impact is totally devastating for the children, young adults and families affected by them. In this chapter I am going to discuss, again through real case studies, therapy and interventions for two patients, one an adolescent, the other a young adult. As we become more knowledgeable about all the different forms of NCD, and the way in which we can treat them with non-pharmacological approaches, we strive to improve quality of life. Due to lifestyle changes in modern society around diet, nutrition and stress, we are witnessing an upsurge in NCD affecting the younger generation. For this reason, clinicians of all disciplines must be skilled in responding to the needs of this cohort.

CASE STUDY

Neuronal Ceroid Lipofuscinoses (NCL) Batten Disease

Neuronal ceroid lipofuscinoses (NCL), or Batten disease, is a metabolic disorder and most common form of NCD. The Batten Disease Family Association in Farnborough estimate that approximately 1 to 3 children are diagnosed with an infantile form of the disease each year and that 7 to 10 children are diagnosed with a late-infantile form of the disease on an annual basis. This means there are between 30 and 60 affected children and young people in the UK. Someone living with Batten disease will experience blindness, complex epilepsy that is difficult to control, myoclonic limb jerks, difficulty sleeping, speech, language and swallowing dysfunction, fine and gross motor skill deterioration, hallucinations, memory loss and behavior that challenges. Mortality occurs between early childhood and young adulthood. As there is no cure, therapy is aimed at improving quality of life for the person diagnosed with the disease and those supporting them through their journey. Over 400 mutations in 13 different genes have been described that lead to the various forms of this disease; thus, each person is affected individually. In this case study I will be focusing on a young man called Sebastian.

Sebastian was 14 years of age when I got involved with his and his family's journey. He had recently been diagnosed with Batten disease after a number of misdiagnoses (this is common with this type of NCD) and the parents had mixed emotions. On the one hand they were pleased they had at last found out what their only child was living with, and on the other they were angry, frustrated and on what they described as an emotional train wreck. Sebastian had not yet developed blindness but experienced many of the other symptoms mentioned above to a mild degree. However, it was his memory and behavioral issues that were causing the biggest impact on both him and his parents, so from a clinical standpoint I needed to address those, along with supporting his parents through their own emotional challenges that presented on a day-to-day basis. Like so many parents, they had no idea that this disease existed or that children could get an NCD in the first place. Figure 12.1 identifies the issues that presented as part of Sebastian's journey.

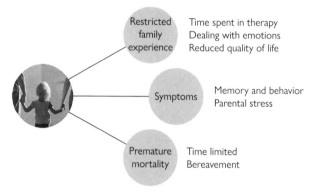

Restricted family experience — Time spent in therapy / Dealing with emotions / Reduced quality of life

Symptoms — Memory and behavior / Parental stress

Premature mortality — Time limited / Bereavement

Figure 12.1 Sebastian's journey

A holistic family approach is required when supporting this type of journey. Everyone is struggling with negative thoughts, feelings and emotions, and though the parents (we shall call them Brenda and Geoff) have been coping with Sebastian's challenges for a number of years, the recent diagnosis has further compacted their mindset. By first identifying the challenges faced by Sebastian and his parents, the clinician is able to put together an appropriate therapy plan with the ultimate aim of improving everyone's quality of life.

Restricted family experience was the term used by Brenda and Geoff when I asked them the first thing that came to mind when they considered their current situation. By breaking that down further, they identified three key areas to be addressed:

- *Time spent in therapy*: For all three, this meant they would miss out on things that other families were doing. For Sebastian, it meant critical time away from his best friend Liam. However, when we discussed the length of time therapy would take, approximately

1 hour three times a week for 6 weeks, and the positive outcomes that would come from therapy, Brenda and Geoff changed their mindset. When I suggested we include Liam in sessions if that was agreeable, Sebastian also had a different view and was looking forward to the sessions. Fortunately, Liam agreed. Following that discussion, we were able to agree a SAP. That was our first breakthrough.

- *Dealing with emotions*: As a family there were shared emotions, and as individuals there were unique ones that needed to be addressed with each person. Everyone was on an emotional rollercoaster, with Brenda and Geoff needing to express their anger and frustration in a structured and supportive manner. Sebastian understood his time was limited and, though he was trying to be positive and upbeat, his true feelings were being expressed through angry outbursts toward his parents, toward himself through self-harm and through the destruction of property. It appeared that Liam was his only calming influence. The inclusion of his best friend in this SAP was critical for a positive, clinical outcome.

- *Reduced quality of life*: Brenda expressed that their quality of life had been compromised for a number of years, and that they hadn't been on a family holiday since their son was 6 years old. Her relationship with Geoff was strained and Sebastian was no longer able to keep up at school. He was requiring more support with everyday tasks and was beginning to have difficulties with his speech and swallowing. The GP, community pediatric team, social worker and other clinicians and therapists were becoming more and more involved, taking up so much time that she and Geoff hardly had a minute alone. I sat down with them and plotted out how much time was spent on clinical matters, GP visits and visits from the social worker. It worked out at approximately 7.5 hours spread over a week, and never at weekends. Having a visual of this timeline showed them all that it was taking up much less time than they first thought. This was our second breakthrough.

Symptoms were a very challenging aspect of this journey, and after looking at all the behavior issues, we agreed the priorities to address. Brenda and Geoff stated that they could handle their son's verbal outbursts but could not bear seeing him self-harm (he would bang his head against the wall or against his own knee) and the destruction of property such as his laptop, desk computer, mobile phone and TV was proving costly. When I started to work with Sebastian it became clear that his frustration at not being able to remember even the basic things was what triggered his aggressive behavior. First, I encouraged him to acknowledge that anger was a natural emotion that we all experience and need to express. Through using the anger ruler method and empty chair therapy, Sebastian was able to learn a different way of expressing his anger, and in addition Liam (and I must point out at this juncture that, at the age of 16, he was extremely mature, intelligent and empathetic, with an amazing insight into Sebastian's plight) also learned these methods in order to act as an aide memoire and greater support to his friend. To address his memory, we placed a large whiteboard in his bedroom where he could choose what was jotted down on it – the important things he wished to remember. His parents or Liam would write these things on the board for him and qualify them with pictures or photos where possible. The myoclonic jerks also caused him frustration and embarrassment so the work here was about focusing on his positive abilities and listening to my recorded relaxation CD whenever his anxiety levels began to rise, a time when the movements intensified. Finally we addressed his fear of the inevitable. This is a very difficult thing for me to do as a clinician, so it has to be 100, if not 1000 times more difficult for the patient/client. He was going to die in the next few years, he knew that, and was angry about it. Active listening and the expression of empathy by the clinician is important, along with warmth, genuineness, honesty and transparency. This helped to build a therapeutic alliance that was mutually beneficial and trusting. It was useful for Sebastian to be able to express these emotions to somebody other than his parents, and he was also seeking permission from somebody to say that it is okay to be upset, bitter and angry at the hand he had been dealt. He found Gestalt (empty chair) therapy to be of the greatest value and over the weeks there was a huge decrease in self-injurious behavior.

Parental stress was also a main challenge, and I addressed it through relationship counseling as well as some 1:1 individual sessions with Brenda and Geoff.

Brenda was a 34-year-old accountant working for a national car sales company. Geoff was 36 and worked as a self-employed IT consultant. They had no other family involvement or support. Financially stable and living in a beautiful home, they both felt that the stress of the situation was beginning to threaten everything they had worked so hard to build, which included their son Sebastian. They were both very devoted parents and couldn't bear the fact that he was experiencing the journey he was living. My aim was to ensure they saw his journey as something they could support him to live well with, and that by focusing on the positives it could be a much smoother journey for all of them. This is a challenge for any clinician as palliative care can be emotionally draining for everyone involved in end-of-life care of a child, and to all intents and purposes, we were all part of that palliative care approach.

One of the biggest issues they were struggling to manage was feelings of guilt. They believed they were responsible for their son's condition, that they had effectively given him a death sentence. These were harsh words to hear, but these were their realities and beliefs. Through the process of joint bereavement counseling, relationship counseling and 1:1 Gestalt therapy, I encouraged them to confront their enemies, mainly fear and guilt, and strip them down to the core. As with most of my patients and clients, the use of Gestalt therapy supports them to achieve the ability to express inner anger, frustrations and other negative emotions in a structured, productive way. As a reminder to clinicians, the principles of Gestalt therapy are organized into five categories, these being proximity, similarity, continuity, closure and connectedness. I used Gestalt to encourage both Brenda and Geoff to focus on the present moment and the adjustments they needed to make as a result of the overall situation. Combined with bereavement and relationship counseling, their mindset began to change and they were able to start building positive images and thoughts that they then put into action with Sebastian. Fritz Perls, who conceived the idea of Gestalt therapy, once said "Nothing changes until it becomes what it is." This resonated with both Brenda and Geoff and it further encouraged them to focus on the present and enjoy every moment of their time with their son.

Premature mortality is inevitable in the case of Sebastian. He realized this and, through my work with him, he began to accept it as best he could. It didn't mean he had let go of the anger he felt that his time was limited and that he wouldn't be able to experience the things his friend would, but he learned new tools to express his anger and a new mindset to see life as it was at the present moment. As a family, they pulled together and supported each other to the maximum, enjoying a quality of life they couldn't imagine prior to clinical intervention and professional support.

A few months after my involvement with the family, Sebastian and his parents, along with Liam and his parents, went to Fuerteventura for 2 weeks and had a fantastic holiday. One week after they returned, Sebastian passed away at home in the company of his parents and Liam. From the input they had received, they were equipped with the tools and mindset to work through their loss and bereavement – tools that would give them the strength to face the rest of their lives.

CASE STUDY

NCD Due to Huntington's Disease

Huntington's disease is a genetic disorder that can present at any age. It leads to progressive breakdown in the brain's neurons and currently has no cure. Patients are affected in different ways and at different stages of the disease. An example of this is where one person has severe chorea and no behavioral challenges, whereas another will present with severe behavioral challenges and very little, or no, chorea.

This disease has a huge impact on the life of the person living with it. When it affects someone in their late teens, that impact is devastating. In this final case study I will discuss an existing client of mine, who we shall call Drake.

Drake was 19 years of age when he was referred to me for psychotherapy in 2017. A few weeks previously he had received news that he was living with juvenile Huntington's disease (JHD), which is a term used for anyone diagnosed under the age of 21. He lived, and continues to live, at home with single mum Sally and 22-year-old girlfriend Jade. He was studying to become a mechanical engineer at his local college and had been making plans to marry Jade and raise a family. The news he received from his GP completely shattered and devastated his entire being and he had been left reeling with shock and total disbelief. Much of the information he had been given at the time had not been absorbed and his mum had been given some literature about the disease, informed about its likely outcomes for her son and was asked to wait for an appointment to see the specialist.

During my first meeting with Drake, Sally and Jade, we formulated the plan you can see in Figure 12.2. This was based on information I received from them and their GP. During the spotlighting meeting, we discussed as much about the situation as possible and were able to prioritize areas to be addressed in order of importance to each of them. It is important to note at this point that Drake had a very close relationship with his mother, who had been a single parent since the untimely death of his father when Drake was only 7 years old. In addition, he had known Jade since he was 10 after she moved in to the same road and attended the same youth club. Every part of this plan is inter-related, and one component would fail as a therapeutic outcome without the inclusion of the other.

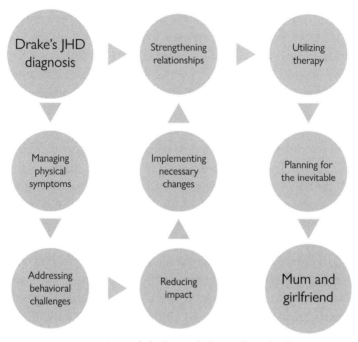

Figure 12.2 Drake's plan, including Sally and Jade

Drake's JHD diagnosis had been delivered like a bombshell. Over the past year or so, everyone had noticed he was different, that he was more clumsy than usual and that his body was beginning to feel rigid. He was less patient and easily got irritated, even at the simplest of things like waiting for the kettle to boil. It had been discovered that his father was likely to be the person who passed on the gene to his son, and Drake had internal rage about that. His mother, Sally, harbored elements of guilt, while Jade was struggling to understand how, and why, this was happening to the man she loved and planned to spend the rest of her life with. There was both misunderstanding and misinformation about JHD after each one of them had been looking on the internet and asking people about the disease.

It was important to start off with a frank discussion about JHD and how it impacts individually on each person. The challenges Drake is facing, and the journey he is on, may be similar to other people but at the same time they are as unique as his own fingerprint or earlobe. It took two full sessions to work through this with the family but once the messages had been driven home, the path was clear to address the other areas that were proving problematic in terms of holding back any progress with the agreed plan.

His internal rage toward his father needed to be expressed, and we did this during a 1:1 session of person centered counseling. The aims here were for Drake to open up and discuss his real feelings toward his father (it transpired that he had never grieved the loss of his father because, at the age of 7, he believed he needed to be strong for his mother), to develop both an increased self-awareness and self-acceptance and to reduce the defensiveness he had created within his own being as a coping strategy. It was the first time he had been able to express such pent-up emotions and this therapeutic approach proved beneficial to Drake. Through our old friend empty chair therapy, he was able to tell his father how he felt about having this genetic curse. At first he was angry toward him; he hated him with a vengeance and was hurt that a father could ever do this to his own son. Eventually, he mellowed and forgave his father as he did not know this was going to happen. Drake stated he had found the closure he needed and we were able to agree that this had now been resolved; that it was time to move on in his own journey through JHD.

My next 1:1 session was with Sally. She had been a teenage mum and brought her son into the world 2 days after her 18th birthday. She was devoted to him and felt blame, shame and guilt for the situation he was experiencing. The focus in this session was to help Sally turn her negative emotions and images into positive ones, so I introduced her to both CBT and NLP. There is nothing anyone can do to change Drake's genetic inheritance or the journey he is due to experience. However, Sally had not passed that gene to her son and she therefore needed to accept the reality of that fact as well as changing her current belief system. One thing that was very helpful post-session was when Drake told his mum she was not to blame, that she could let go of that belief and instead focus on completing the law degree she started with the Open University 3 years earlier. He reinforced the fact that he would be so proud of her if she did that. With a further 1:1 session using hypnotherapy to help Sally let go of the negative beliefs and emotions, we were able to remove the brambles that had served as a barrier to positively supporting Drake along his new journey.

Initially, Jade stated she didn't need any 1:1 therapy but was happy to be present and supportive at any further sessions I had with Drake.

Managing physical symptoms was the role of the GP and specialist but also needed addressing in terms of how they affected Drake. At my time of input, the symptoms affecting Drake were rigidity, mild dystonia (these are muscle contractions that cause repetitive or twisting movements), bradykinesia (these are slow movements) and cognitive deficit (in Drake's case, his immediate memory was affected along with regular, but not always, disorientation in time and place). Though there are medicines to help with chorea, Drake didn't want to take them as he was managing those symptoms through meditation and yoga, which he had practiced since the age of 15. I taught him how to further manage his symptoms through self-hypnosis, another technique he was familiar with. These strategies also proved useful with his cognitive deficits, though it was these that led to his behavioral challenges.

Addressing behavioral challenges that caused problems for all of them was an agreed action. These were triggered by Drake's cognitive deficits in combination with mild depression and general anxiety disorder. He would get frustrated and throw objects across the room, shout, swear and kick the wall. I found that an eclectic combination of CBT and hypno-psychotherapy helped to change the way in which he thought about his cognitive deficits. By using the STOPP sheet and anger management ruler, Drake took both control of and responsibility for his behavior. STOPP refers to the following:

- Stop.

- Take a breath.

- Observe – describe the feelings, images, thoughts, body sensations and triggers.

- Pull back/put in some perspective. What's the bigger picture? Take the helicopter view. Is this fact or fiction? Is there another way of looking at the situation?

- Practice what works – what is the best thing to do right now? For me, for others, for the situation.

Reducing impact of the diagnosis and prognosis affecting all their plans for the future was critical. It shaped who they were becoming and was seen as one of the many enemies that would destroy them all if they allowed it to do so. Therapy and support within the family infrastructure was paramount if the journey was to be as comfortable as possible. By reaching out to a number of distant family members they realized they could expand their support network (just as an aside, Drake discovered a relative he never knew existed, and over the months their friendship blossomed and proved invaluable).

Implementing necessary changes had to be made on both an individual and family level. Life for Drake, his mother and girlfriend was never going to be the same again. There would need to be adjustments in many areas, including mindset and the physical environment. Thinking about those things helped create a plan that was flexible enough to change as and when needed.

Strengthening relationships that had been strained of late was a shared objective. Each person was dealing with the current situation in their own individual way, utilizing their own coping strategies to get through each day. However, one thing that remained constant was the love and affection they clearly felt for each other. This closeness was one of the main reasons for successful outcomes from therapy.

Utilizing therapy was necessary in order to equip Drake, Sally and Jade with the tools they would need for the coming months and years. As we have seen, various therapies were helpful to Drake and his mum, and after a few weeks Jade asked for a 1:1 session. She was struggling with the images of Drake as he deteriorates – she had looked on the internet and seen images of people in the very end stages of the disease and it had left an imprint. I decided a technique known as accelerated resolution therapy (ART) would be the most suitable modality of psychotherapy to address this issue. This is a relatively straightforward and swift therapy that uses relaxing eye movements and a technique referred to as voluntary memory and image replacement. ART was developed in 2008 by Laney Rosenzweig, a marriage and family therapist. Since 2015, the National Registry of Evidence-based Programs and Practices have officially recognized ART as an evidence-based practice. Use of ART would change the way in which Jade's negative images were stored in her brain. The outcome was that those images no longer triggered the strong emotions and reactions of inconsolable crying, shaking and panic that they had led to prior to the therapy.

Planning for the inevitable had to be included in the work I was doing with the family. Drake had a life expectancy of between 10 and 15 years, though there are no guarantees. Over time, his cognitive and physical function will deteriorate as JHD is neurodegenerative. Toward the end of my input with the family, they had a positive mindset with the skills and tools required to face whatever came their way. Drake intended to live life to the full and cram as much as possible into those years, including marriage. As part of their plan, he and Jade were to be married toward the end of 2017. They booked their honeymoon and Sally was occupied making wedding plans with the couple.

Mum and girlfriend must have the ability to support each other as Drake's journey progresses into its severest form and end stages. As such, they learned as much accurate information about the disease as possible. They learned about strategies they could use to support Drake along each stage of the journey and accessed all the necessary human and financial resources available.

My role was to ensure Drake and his family were equipped with the tools necessary to enjoy the best quality of life possible. I was confident that I had done that. At the time of writing in mid-2018, Drake and Jade are happily married and he now has a very close friendship with a cousin he discovered as part of my input with the family. Sally is close to completing her law degree and is looking forward to making her son proud when she is awarded her degree. Together, they have a difficult and challenging journey ahead, but all of them now have the strength to make the journey as positive as can be.

Conclusion

This book has discussed, in depth, ways in which clinicians (and others) can enhance the quality of life of people living with an NCD and those supporting their unique journey.

My intention has been to demonstrate that a diagnosis of Alzheimer's disease or another primary NCD is no longer all doom and gloom. On the contrary, if the correct approach is adopted, we can have a positive impact on those we serve.

As we continue to learn about the function of the brain and the power of neuroplasticity, while unraveling the mysteries of the mind, we begin to understand ways in which we can achieve rementia through non-pharmacological interventions. This is not to say medication won't have a role to play at some point, but this must be as part of an overall collaborative approach. When providing clinical interventions to seniors, it is very difficult to avoid polypharmacy due to the fact that the clinician may be managing multiple morbidities; for example, mixed dementia, heart disease and diabetes.

Through the application of the therapies discussed, in conjunction with the models identified, we can reduce fear and anxiety, enhance communication, empower individuals and go a long way to extinguishing (now there's an old behaviorists' term!) behaviors that impact negatively on the life of everyone experiencing their unique journey.

If each and every one of us sets out at the start of the day with the mindset that we will turn someone's frown into a smile, the law of collective consciousness means our impact will reach a worldwide audience!

If we educate the youth of today on brain health, lifestyle and diet and nutrition, we can help them reduce their risk of developing an NCD later in life. By adopting the DTS-VADRA2016, clinicians can help adults, young and old, to reduce their risks of developing vascular dementia and Alzheimer's disease.

Finally, someone in the UK is diagnosed with dementia every 3 minutes. That's 480 people every single day. I believe we have both a clinical and moral duty to be proactive in strategies that reduce this number, and reactive through true person centered therapies with those who have developed a cognitive change.

Thank you for reading this book and for the support you provide to individuals as they embark on their journey.

References

All Party Political Group on Dementia (APPG) (2008) "Always a last resort: Inquiry into the prescription of antipsychotic drugs to people with dementia in care homes." Alzheimer's Society, London.

Alzheimer's Society (2007) "Home from home: A report highlighting opportunities for improving standards of dementia care in care homes." Alzheimer's Society, London.

American Psychiatric Association (1998) "American Psychiatric Association practice guideline on dementia." *American Family Physician, 57*(2), 366–375.

American Psychiatric Association (2013) *Diagnostic and Statistical Manual of Mental Disorders*, fifth edition (DSM-5). APA, Washington, DC.

Asher, M. (1999) *Body Language.* Carlton, London.

Bandler, R. and Grinder, J. (1975) *The Structure of Magic: A Book about Language and Therapy*, vol. 1. Science and Behavior, Palo Alto, CA.

Burns, A., Guthrie, E., Marino-Francis, F., Busby, C., Morris, J., Russell, E., Margison, F., Lennon, S. and Byrne, J. (2005) "Brief psychotherapy in Alzheimer's disease: Randomised controlled trial." *British Journal of Psychiatry 188*, 192.

Cheston, R., Jones, K. and Gillard, J. (2003) "Group psychotherapy and people with dementia." *Aging and Mental Health, 7*(6), 452–461.

Clark, D.M. (2011) "Implementing NICE guidelines for the psychological treatment of depression and anxiety disorders: The IAPT experience." *International Review of Psychiatry, 23*(4), 318–327.

Department of Health (DoH) (2009) *Living Well with Dementia: A National Dementia Strategy*. Department of Health, London.

Duff, S.C. and Nightingale, D.J. (2005) "The efficacy of hypnosis in changing the quality of life in patients with dementia. A pilot-study evaluation." *European Journal of Clinical Hypnosis, 6*(2), 20–29.

Duff, S.C. and Nightingale, D.J. (2006) "Long term outcomes of hypnosis in changing the quality of life in patients with dementia." *European Journal of Clinical Hypnosis, 7*(1), 2–8.

Duff, S.C. and Nightingale, D.J. (2007) "Alternative approaches to supporting people with dementia: Enhancing quality of life through hypnosis." *Alzheimer's Care Today, 8*(4), 321–331.

Duffy, M. (2002) "Strategies for working with women with dementia." In *Psychotherapy for Counselling with Older Women: Cross Cultural, Family and End of Life Issues* (eds F.K. Rotman and C.M. Brody). Springer, New York, pp. 175–194.

Estruch, R., Ros, E., Salas-Salvado, J. and Covas, M.I. (2013) "Primary prevention of cardiovascular disease with a Mediterranean diet." *New England Journal of Medicine, 368*, 1279–1290.

Fossey, J., Ballard, C., Juszczak, E., James, I., Alder, N., Jacoby, R. and Howard, R. (2006) "Effect of enhanced psychosocial care on antipsychotic use in nursing home residents with severe dementia: Cluster randomised trial." *BMJ, 332*(7544), 756–761.

Ivanis, S. (1992) "Brockhall/Calderstones Department of Clinical Psychology report on the effects of residential relocation." NHS, Whalley, UK.

Kaiser Stearns, A. (1984) *Living Through Personal Crisis*. Thomas More Press, USA.

King, I. (1981) *A Theory for Nursing: Systems, Concepts, Process*. Wiley, Chicago, IL.

Kitwood, T. (1997) *Dementia Reconsidered: The Person Comes First (Reconsidering Ageing)*. Open University Press, Milton Keynes.

Knapp, M., Thorgrimsen, L., Patel, A., Spector, A., Hallam, A., Woods, B. and Orrell, M. (2006) "Cognitive stimulation therapy for people with dementia: Cost-effectiveness analysis (randomized controlled trial)." *British Journal of Psychiatry, 188*, 574–580.

Kolb, A.Y. and Kolb, D.A. (2012) "Experiential learning theory." In *Encyclopedia of the Sciences of Learning* (ed. N.M. Seel). Springer, New York, pp. 1215–1219.

Maslow, A. (1943) "A theory of human motivation." *Psychological Review, 50*(4), 370–396.

Nightingale, D. (2011) "Montessori success for people living with dementia." *Journal of Dementia Care, 19*(2), 36–38.

Norman-Haignere, S. (2015) "Music in the Brain." *MIT News*, December 16.

O'Brien, J. (1989) *What's Worth Working For? Leadership for Better Quality Human Services*. Center on Human Policy, Syracuse University, Syracuse, NY.

Ott, A., Stolk, R.P., Hofman, A., van Harskamp, F., Grobbee, D.E. and Breteler, M.M.B. (1996) "Association of Diabetes Mellitus and Dementia: The Rotterdam study." *Diabetalogia, 39*, 1392–1397.

Padesky, C.A. (1993) "Socratic questioning: Changing minds or guiding discovery?" Keynote address delivered at the European Congress of Behavioural and Cognitive Therapies, London.

Pezzati, R., Molteni, V., Bani, M., Settanta, C., Grazia Di Maggio, M., Villa, I., Poletti, B. and Ardito, R.B. (2014) "Can doll therapy preserve or promote attachment in people with cognitive, behavioural, and emotional problems? A pilot study in institutionalized patients with dementia." *Frontiers in Psychology, 5*, 342.

Reber, S. and Reber, E. (2009) *The Penguin Dictionary of Psychology*. Penguin, London.

Reisberg, B., Ferris, S.H., de Leon, M.J. and Crook, T. (1982) "The Global Deterioration Scale for assessment of primary degenerative dementia." *The American Journal of Psychiatry, 139*(9), 1136–1139.

Riemersma-van der Lek, R.F., Swab, D.F., Twisk, J., Hol, E.M., Hoogendijk, W.J. and Van Someren, E.J. (2008) "Effect of bright light and melatonin on cognitive and noncognitive function in elderly residents of group care facilities." *JAMA, 299*(22), 2642–2655.

Simon, E.P. and Canonico, M.M. (2001) "Use of hypnosis in controlling lumbar puncture distress in an adult needle-phobic dementia patient." *International Journal of Clinical Hypnosis, 49*(1), 56–67.

Snowdon, D. (2001) *Aging with Grace: What the Nun Study Teaches us About Leading Longer, Healthier, and More Meaningful Lives.* Penguin, London.

Spiegal, H. and Spiegal, D. (1978) *Trance and Treatment: Clinical Uses of Hypnosis.* Basic Books, New York.

van Hoof, J., Kort, H.S., van Waarde, H. and Blom, M.M. (2010) "Environmental interventions and the design of houses for older adults with dementia." *American Journal of Alzheimer's Disease and Other Dementias, 25*(3), 202–232.

Wang, J., Ho, L., Zhao, Z., Seror, I., Humala, N., Dickstein, D.L., Thiyagarajan, M., Percival, S.S., Talcott, S.T. and Pasinetti, G.M. (2006) "Moderate consumption of cabernet sauvignon attenuates Abeta neuropathology in a mouse model of Alzheimer's disease." *FASEB Journal, 20*(13), 2313–2320.

Welden, S. and Yesavage, J.A. (1982) "Behavioural improvement with relocation training in senile dementia." *Clinical Gerontology, 1*, 45–49.

World Health Organization (2016) *International Statistical Classification of Diseases and Related Health Problems*, 10th edition (ICD-10). WHO, Geneva, Switzerland.

Zablotsky, B., Black, L.I., Maenner, M.J., Schieve, L.A. and Blumberg, S.J. (2015) "Estimated prevalence of autism and other developmental disabilities following questionnaire changes in the 2014 National Health Interview Survey." *National Health Statistics Report, 13*(87), 1–20.

Index